AF750876

Exploring AI in Pain Research and Management

Marco Cascella

Exploring AI in Pain Research and Management

Springer

Marco Cascella
Unit of Anesthesiology, Intensive Care Medicine and Pain Medicine
University of Salerno
Baronissi, Salerno, Italy

ISBN 978-3-031-78832-1 ISBN 978-3-031-78833-8 (eBook)
https://doi.org/10.1007/978-3-031-78833-8

© The Editor(s) (if applicable) and The Author(s), under exclusive license to Springer Nature Switzerland AG 2024
This work is subject to copyright. All rights are solely and exclusively licensed by the Publisher, whether the whole or part of the material is concerned, specifically the rights of translation, reprinting, reuse of illustrations, recitation, broadcasting, reproduction on microfilms or in any other physical way, and transmission or information storage and retrieval, electronic adaptation, computer software, or by similar or dissimilar methodology now known or hereafter developed.
The use of general descriptive names, registered names, trademarks, service marks, etc. in this publication does not imply, even in the absence of a specific statement, that such names are exempt from the relevant protective laws and regulations and therefore free for general use.
The publisher, the authors and the editors are safe to assume that the advice and information in this book are believed to be true and accurate at the date of publication. Neither the publisher nor the authors or the editors give a warranty, expressed or implied, with respect to the material contained herein or for any errors or omissions that may have been made. The publisher remains neutral with regard to jurisdictional claims in published maps and institutional affiliations.

This Springer imprint is published by the registered company Springer Nature Switzerland AG
The registered company address is: Gewerbestrasse 11, 6330 Cham, Switzerland

If disposing of this product, please recycle the paper.

Foreword

Pain is one of the most devastating symptoms for our patients and their loved ones. Unfortunately, there has been very limited progress in our ability to assess and manage severe and persistent pain.

One of the main limitations has been the lack of reliable tools for the assessment and monitoring of this complex multidimensional symptom.

In the last 2 years, we have seen an explosion of literature on the potential role of artificial intelligence in medicine. One of the main barriers to integrating the fields of AI and pain medicine has been the very limited understanding that experts from both fields have about each other's discipline. Dr. Cascella's outstanding book comes to the rescue of both pain medicine and AI experts.

This book provides a first introduction to artificial intelligence. Many clinicians, including myself, will be surprised and inspired by this progress. This book discusses, in a user-friendly format, all the different modalities of AI and ways in which it might assist in the understanding of pain.

The second part of this book is a sophisticated discussion of all aspects of the production and transmission of pain at multiple levels. The complex interaction between sensorial, cognitive, and emotional brain regions is discussed in a way that helps understand how AI might benefit from the current knowledge in the development of models.

The third part is, in my view, the most exciting. It addresses all the possible dimensions of automatic pain assessment, from facial expressions to complex cardiovascular and neurological assessments. This book discusses how well AI can integrate all these multiple dimensions to conduct assessments over time and assist clinicians and patients in their decision-making.

The last part of this book addresses the way AI and pain medicine have the capability to completely change patient care. The creation of reliable predictive models for the main clinical outcomes, such as pain relief or the development of opioid use disorder, has the potential to improve pain management everywhere very soon.

This book should be read by all clinicians, including physicians, nurses, pharmacists, and psychologists, who are involved in the care of patients with pain, as well as for experts in artificial intelligence in medicine.

The single-author nature of this book makes it particularly consistent and much easier to read. I am convinced that readers will enjoy this book just as much as I did. I am grateful to Dr. Cascella for this enormous effort, which will help so many patients in years to come.

Palliative Care and Rehabilitation Medicine
University of Texas MD Anderson Cancer Center
Houston, TX, USA

Eduardo Bruera

Preface

There is no doubt that the rapid development and widespread application of artificial intelligence (AI) are impacting our daily lives and society, including the fields of medicine and healthcare. Furthermore, the intersection of AI and pain research and management is a field of study with vast potential. However, the successful application of AI in clinical settings requires a deep understanding of both the technological and clinical landscapes as well. The primary challenge lies in applying AI to the complex issue of pain. In various clinical scenarios, AI can greatly benefit from utilizing objective data. For instance, imaging data or those from patients scheduled for surgical interventions can be "easily" analyzed by AI to enhance assessment and management strategies. These dynamics cannot be applied *tout court* to the study of pain phenomena.

Automatic pain assessment (APA) is a broad term used to indicate the objective study of pain. Significantly, we have a range of techniques for APA that enable the study of pain through various biosignals and imaging methods. Each method provides unique insights into the neural and physiological responses to pain. However, despite their potential, the practical application of these techniques faces significant challenges. The limitations of APA often stem from the complexity of pain mechanisms, the variability in individual responses, and the influence of external factors. Significantly, pain is expressed in highly individual ways, and there is no straightforward correlation between behavioral cues and the intensity or quality of pain. This holds even in controlled laboratory experiments where pain is induced in healthy subjects. As a result, significant effort is required to develop a "gold standard" for assessing the effectiveness of pain detection methods.

Therefore, while APA methods offer valuable data, their practical results can sometimes be insurmountable in clinical practice. For example, regarding biosignals, since too many factors influence the sympathetic and parasympathetic systems, it would be impossible to define a single technique that better objectively characterizes the processes of pain. The same limitation applies to other APA strategies. On these bases, it seems that an integrated approach using multiple techniques could be a promising strategy. Anesthesiologists acknowledge that by tracking changes in physiological signals like skin conductance and heart rate, reliable indices for pain assessment, such as the analgesia nociception index, have been developed. However, the autonomic nervous system, and the balance between the sympathetic and parasympathetic branches, can respond to factors other than the noxious stimulus. Thus, physiological measurements using nociception indices are most effective in controlled environments, like operating rooms, where the patient is unconscious, and these metrics provide the only means of monitoring pain. In other settings, a more comprehensive, multicomponent approach is required. It is mandatory to face the multiple aspects that collectively shape the complex pain phenomenon.

However, the questions remain: which combination of techniques should be used, in which patients, and in what context? The research questions are endless. More importantly, to be exact, these methods should be classified as *stress detection strategies*, as they can detect shifts in the balance of the autonomic nervous system components. However, this does not necessarily indicate nociception or pain.

In this complex landscape, the utilization of AI and a multiprofessional collaboration involving clinicians, computer scientists, bioengineers, and other researchers could be the key to crossing the AI chasm, ultimately unlocking new insights.

This book aims to provide clinicians, computer scientists, and engineers with a clinical and translational perspective on AI in pain research and management, emphasizing the importance of interdisciplinary collaboration and the challenges of data quality and integration. This book is structured into four comprehensive chapters. The first chapter introduces fundamental concepts of AI, tailored for clinicians. It covers essential topics such as machine learning, neural networks, and natural language processing, demystifying technical jargon to bridge the knowledge gap between clinical practice and AI technology. The chapter "Research in Automatic Pain Assessment" delves into current research on APA, exploring innovative methodologies and technologies. It highlights advancements in facial expression analysis, speech analysis, and different physiological signal processing (biosignals). The research aims to develop integrated models, in other words, frameworks for a "Pain Holter," namely systems for continuous and non-invasive monitoring and support for therapy.

AI is not limited to APA; predictive and generative models have been developed for a wide range of applications. Another chapter focuses on the practical applications of AI within different clinical settings. It discusses real-world implementations, such as AI-driven pain management tools, predictive analytics for treatment outcomes, and personalized pain therapy, demonstrating the transformative potential of AI in enhancing patient care. Finally, a chapter is devoted to offering a clinical and translational perspective aimed at computer scientists and researchers from different fields. It suggests ways to apply AI expertise in developing effective pain management solutions. This chapter aims to give non-clinicians a foundational understanding while keeping domain-specific terminology to a minimum. The key connection between clinical researchers and computer scientists or bioengineers lies in the data collection interface used. It is the cornerstone of each APA framework. Therefore, the chapter includes insights into developing a dashboard for gathering multidimensional data. From these premises, a research framework is ultimately proposed. Although there is significant overlap between methods used for animals and humans, factors such as ethical considerations, communication challenges, and physiological differences necessitate a distinct review of APA in rodents and other animals.

I hope that expert readers will find valuable insights and ideas for developing or enhancing their frameworks. I welcome any feedback on inaccuracies or suggestions for improvement. This field is still emerging, and even a book can be an opportunity to build fruitful collaborations. To non-expert readers, I apologize if the material is tedious, but I have made every effort to present it as clearly as possible.

For acknowledgment, Grammarly (Grammarly, Inc.) and GPT-4 were used for language improvements and general manuscript revision. After using these tools, the author reviewed and edited the content as needed and takes full responsibility for the publication's content.

Baronissi, Salerno, Italy Marco Cascella

Contents

1 Introduction

Pain is one of the most prevalent symptoms requiring medical intervention. It is a complex stressful, subjective, and multidimensional experience. While acute (e.g., post-injury or postoperative) pain serves as an essential alarm signal, triggering adaptive and homeostatic responses, chronic pain is a multifaceted phenomenon that encompasses biological, psychological, and social issues [1]. Characterizing acute and chronic pain forms adds another layer of complexity, both temporally and as their underlying pathophysiology [2]. The transition from acute to chronic pain, along with its clinical manifestations, is a critical area of study, and several aspects need to be better elucidated. For example, some forms of chronic pain emerge without preceding acute pain phases [3, 4].

Furthermore, it must be emphasized that nociception and pain (the reported experience) are separate processes. The advancement of computational methods in recent decades has enabled the creation of models that enhance our understanding of pain mechanisms [5]. Nociception refers to the physiological mechanism by which our body detects and responds to potentially harmful stimuli or noxious input. In other words, it is the neural process of encoding noxious stimuli. Schematically, nociception is essentially the body's sensory system aimed at alerting for potential tissue damage or injury. This process involves the transmission of signals from specialized nerve receptors (nociceptors) to the central nervous system, where the information is processed [6]. For research purposes in the field of robot perception, artificial nociceptors have also been developed. These receptors are infrared proximity sensors embedded within the robot's "artificial skin," designed to respond to various types of stimuli [7].

Therefore, pain involves the perception and interpretation of these signals by the brain, encompassing not only the sensory aspect but also the emotional and cognitive dimensions [8]. On these premises, pain is influenced by a range of factors, including the nature of the stimulus, biological aspects, and psychological and social elements. These varying influences can interfere with accurately assessing pain, making objective measurement more difficult.

© The Author(s), under exclusive license to Springer Nature Switzerland AG 2024

M. Cascella, *Exploring AI in Pain Research and Management*,
https://doi.org/10.1007/978-3-031-78833-8_1

In this highly complex scenario, having reliable diagnostic reference points is crucial for structuring effective therapeutic pathways. Clinical examination and detailed patient history should complement patient-reported data. However, the biopsychosocial complexities of pain and its emotional content make subjective data potentially misleading, leading to undertreatment or overtreatment [9].

An emerging approach still under research focuses on automatic pain assessment (APA). This term refers to a set of methodologies that study the objective components related to pain, such as biosignal responses and observable behaviors, including facial expressions of pain and speech analyses. These strategies can be explored by implementing artificial intelligence (AI) techniques [10]. AI can analyze vast amounts of biosignal data, identifying patterns and correlations that might be imperceptible to human clinicians. For example, machine learning algorithms can be trained to recognize specific physiological responses to different pain levels, providing a more objective and consistent measure of pain intensity [11]. Moreover, computational language analyses can be implemented for pain [12] and emotion recognition [13]. Additionally, computer vision seems to be a suitable tool for investigating pain-related facial expressions [14].

Nevertheless, while APA methods have the potential to offer more objective insights into pain intensity, it is crucial to acknowledge their limitations. These mostly include the lack of high-quality validation studies, uncertainty about which parameters should be implemented in different settings, and technical issues such as timing of utilization. Consequently, a comprehensive pain assessment approach should ideally combine both subjective self-reporting and objective measures to provide a more holistic understanding of pain experiences and enable better-informed pain management strategies [15].

Objective pain diagnosis is not the only application of AI in pain medicine. The potential applications of predictive and generative models are multiple and range from the diagnosis of complex clinical conditions, such as fibromyalgia [16], to the definition of clinical trajectories [17, 18], to clinical monitoring processes using dedicated instruments, also in the telehealth field [19]. The goal is to provide personalized treatments tailored to each patient and their specific pain condition.

Thanks to the availability of training on a vast amount of data, generative AI models are in a full evolutionary phase. Natural language processing technologies such as large language models (LLMs) appear to be an incredible resource for chatbot structure and dialogue tools [20]. In pain medicine, they can also support clinicians in analyzing texts and aiding decision-making [21]. Multimodal LLMs such as GPT-4 Vision, Gemini 1.0 Pro Vision, and Claude 3 can process multiple forms of data, such as text, images, and audio, and perform tasks like image captioning, visual question answering, and generating text descriptions from images or videos. The initial efforts toward medical diagnoses are underway [22].

This list of AI applications in pain medicine is quite incomplete. For instance, gamification processes aimed at assistance, education, and training [23], along with the various applications of extended reality [24], are just additional examples. Furthermore, AI systems applied to pain assessment can also be developed to identify pain in vulnerable individuals such as infants [25] or those with communication difficulties [26]. Additionally, following translational perspectives, research is also being conducted on automatic pain detection in animals [27].

The real challenge in the field of AI in pain medicine lies in integrating various research strategies and professionals. This complex process requires collaboration between clinicians who specialize in pain management and possess a background in computer science (expert domain), as well as diverse technical professionals who can tackle different research challenges. These professionals include, for example, experts in computer vision for image processing, natural language processing specialists for linguistic analysis, bioengineers for biosignals investigations, and others. It is the responsibility of the domain expert to synthesize these diverse skills into a cohesive research program. Nevertheless, this program is often difficult to define in advance and must dynamically adapt to the inevitable progress and setbacks encountered along the way [25]. Probably, it is the most intriguing aspect of this journey.

References

1. Rahman S, Kidwai A, Rakhamimova E, Elias M, Caldwell W, Bergese SD. Clinical diagnosis and treatment of chronic pain. Diagnostics. 2023;13:3689. https://doi.org/10.3390/diagnostics13243689.
2. Cohen SP, Vase L, Hooten WM. Chronic pain: an update on burden, best practices, and new advances. Lancet. 2021;397(10289):2082–97. https://doi.org/10.1016/S0140-6736(21)00393-7.
3. Clauw DJ. From fibrositis to fibromyalgia to nociplastic pain: how rheumatology helped get us here and where do we go from here? Ann Rheum Dis. 2024;83(11):1421–7. https://doi.org/10.1136/ard-2023-225327.
4. Kaplan CM, Kelleher E, Irani A, Schrepf A, Clauw DJ, Harte SE. Deciphering nociplastic pain: clinical features, risk factors and potential mechanisms. Nat Rev Neurol. 2024;20(6):347–63. https://doi.org/10.1038/s41582-024-00966-8.
5. Lang VA, Lundh T, Ortiz-Catalan M. Mathematical and computational models for pain: a systematic review. Pain Med. 2021;22:2806–17. https://doi.org/10.1093/pm/pnab177.
6. Kutafina E, Becker S, Namer B. Measuring pain and nociception: through the glasses of a computational scientist. Transdisciplinary overview of methods. Front Netw Physiol. 2023;3:1099282. https://doi.org/10.3389/fnetp.2023.1099282.
7. L'Haridon L, Cañamero L. The effects of stress and predation on pain perception in robots. In: 2023 11th international conference on affective computing and intelligent interaction (ACII), Cambridge, MA, USA, 2023. pp. 1–8. https://doi.org/10.1109/ACII59096.2023.10388190.
8. Treede R-D, Rief W, Barke A, Aziz Q, Bennett MI, Benoliel R, et al. Chronic pain as a symptom or a disease: the IASP classification of chronic pain for the international classification of diseases (ICD-11). Pain. 2019;160:19–27.
9. Nicholas MK. The biopsychosocial model of pain 40 years on: time for a reappraisal? Pain. 2022;163:S3–S14. https://doi.org/10.1097/j.pain.0000000000002654.
10. Cascella M, Schiavo D, Cuomo A, Ottaiano A, Perri F, Patrone R, Migliarelli S, Bignami EG, Vittori A, Cutugno F. Artificial intelligence for automatic pain assessment: research methods and perspectives. Pain Res Manag. 2023;2013:6018736. https://doi.org/10.1155/2023/6018736.
11. Lötsch J, Ultsch A, Mayer B, Kringel D. Artificial intelligence and machine learning in pain research: a data scientometric analysis. Pain Rep. 2022;7(6):e1044. https://doi.org/10.1097/PR9.0000000000001044.

12. Albashayreh A, Bandyopadhyay A, Zeinali N, Zhang M, Fan W, Gilbertson White S. Natural language processing accurately differentiates cancer symptom information in electronic health record narratives. JCO Clin Cancer Inform. 2024;8:e2300235. https://doi.org/10.1200/CCI.23.00235.
13. Machová K, Szabóova M, Paralič J, Mičko J. Detection of emotion by text analysis using machine learning. Front Psychol. 2023;14:1190326. https://doi.org/10.3389/fpsyg.2023.1190326.
14. D'Antoni F, Russo F, Ambrosio L, Vollero L, Vadalà G, Merone M, Papalia R, Denaro V. Artificial intelligence and computer vision in low back pain: a systematic review. Int J Environ Res Public Health. 2021;18(20):10909. https://doi.org/10.3390/ijerph182010909.
15. Cascella M, Di Gennaro P, Crispo A, Vittori A, Petrucci E, Sciorio F, Marinangeli F, Ponsiglione AM, Romano M, Ovetta C, Ottaiano A, Sabbatino F, Perri F, Piazza O, Coluccia S. Advancing the integration of biosignal-based automated pain assessment methods into a comprehensive model for addressing cancer pain. BMC Palliat Care. 2024;23(1):198. https://doi.org/10.1186/s12904-024-01526-z.
16. Venerito V, Iannone F. Large language model-driven sentiment analysis for facilitating fibromyalgia diagnosis. RMD Open. 2024;10(2):e004367. https://doi.org/10.1136/rmdopen-2024-004367.
17. Lin T, Peng S, Lu S, Fu S, Zeng D, Li J, et al. Prediction of knee pain improvement over two years for knee osteoarthritis using a dynamic nomogram based on MRI-derived radiomics: a proof-of-concept study. Osteoarthr Cartil. 2023;31(2):267–78.
18. Guan B, Liu F, Mizaian AH, Demehri S, Samsonov A, Guermazi A, et al. Deep learning approach to predict pain progression in knee osteoarthritis. Skeletal Radiol. 2022;51(2):363–73.
19. Cascella M, Schiavo D, Grizzuti M, Romano MC, Coluccia S, Bimonte S, Cuomo A. Implementation of a hybrid care model for telemedicine-based cancer pain management at the Cancer Center of Naples, Italy: a cohort study. In Vivo. 2023;37(1):385–92. https://doi.org/10.21873/invivo.13090.
20. Cascella M, Semeraro F, Montomoli J, Bellini V, Piazza O, Bignami E. The breakthrough of large language models release for medical applications: 1-year timeline and perspectives. J Med Syst. 2024;48(1):22. https://doi.org/10.1007/s10916-024-02045-3.
21. Yilmaz Muluk S, Olcucu N. Comparative analysis of artificial intelligence platforms: ChatGPT-3.5 and GoogleBard in identifying red flags of low back pain. Cureus. 2024;16(7):e63580. https://doi.org/10.7759/cureus.63580.
22. Kaczmarczyk R, Wilhelm TI, Martin R, Roos J. Evaluating multimodal AI in medical diagnostics. NPJ Digit Med. 2024;7(1):205. https://doi.org/10.1038/s41746-024-01208-3.
23. Cascella M, Cascella A, Monaco F, Shariff MN. Envisioning gamification in anesthesia, pain management, and critical care: basic principles, integration of artificial intelligence, and simulation strategies. J Anesth Analg Crit Care. 2024;3(1):33. https://doi.org/10.1186/s44158-023-00118-2.
24. Aristidou A, Jena R, Topol EJ. Bridging the chasm between AI and clinical implementation. Lancet. 2022;399:620.
25. Gholami B, Haddad WM, Tannenbaum AR. Relevance vector machine learning for neonate pain intensity assessment using digital imaging. IEEE Trans Biomed Eng. 2010;57(6):1457–66. https://doi.org/10.1109/TBME.2009.2039214.
26. Smith E, Storch EA, Vahia I, et al. Affective computing for late-life mood and cognitive disorders. Front Psychiatry. 2021;12:782183. https://doi.org/10.3389/fpsyt.2021.782183.782183.
27. Andresen N, Wöllhaf M, Hohlbaum K, Lewejohann L, Hellwich O, Thöne-Reineke C, Belik V. Towards a fully automated surveillance of well-being status in laboratory mice using deep learning: starting with facial expression analysis. PLoS One. 2020;15(4):e0228059. https://doi.org/10.1371/journal.pone.0228059.

Basic Knowledge of AI for Clinicians

2

2.1 Brief History of Artificial Intelligence

It is difficult to trace the history of such a complex discipline that intertwines multiple fields of study, from mathematics to statistics to computer science. Although the foundations for AI development were probably established by René Descartes (1596–1659) and Thomas Hobbes (1588–1679) in the seventeenth century, ideally, the birth of artificial intelligence (AI) is traced back to the mid-twentieth century. One of the first significant steps came in 1943 when the neurophysiologist and cybernetician Warren McCulloch (1898–1969) and the computational neuroscientist Walter Pitts (1923–1969) proposed the first model of an artificial neuron [1], which was fundamental for the subsequent development of neural networks. The McCulloch-Pitts neuron provided a simplified representation of how a biological neuron functions in the human brain, establishing the idea that complex thought processes could be represented by simple logical operations on binary numbers [2]. In 1950, Alan Turing, who is considered a founding father of AI, established the theoretical basis for AI research with his seminal paper "Computing Machinery and Intelligence" published on Mind [3]. The English genius introduced the famous Turing Test as a criterion for evaluating a machine's intelligence. This concept stimulated extensive debates on whether machines could achieve human-like intelligence and has remained a foundational concept in AI. Turing's work questioned the philosophical underpinnings of machine intelligence and posited that if a machine could carry on a conversation indistinguishable from a human, it could be said to think. However, already previously, in the 1930s, Turing had dealt with computational processes. In 1936, he proposed the computational machine (now termed as "Turing machine"). It was not a physical machine but only a theoretical model of a machine capable of executing computable sequences [2, 4]. Significantly, the experiments from McCulloch and Pitts were based on the Turing machine.

The term "artificial intelligence" was coined by John McCarthy (1927–2011) during the famous Conference at Dartmouth College (New Hampshire, United

© The Author(s), under exclusive license to Springer Nature Switzerland AG 2024
M. Cascella, *Exploring AI in Pain Research and Management*, https://doi.org/10.1007/978-3-031-78833-8_2

States), in 1956. This event is considered the official birth of AI as a distinct field of study. The Conference brought together key figures in AI, including Marvin Minsky, Nathaniel Rochester, and Claude Shannon, setting the stage for future AI research. McCarthy also played a key role in developing perception algorithms, designing the programming language family Lisp, and promoting different fields of AI research. Therefore, he is recognized as one of the founders of symbolic AI and programming [5].

Since a single neuron cannot organize a cognitive process, a functional structure with interconnections is necessary. In 1957, the American psychologist Frank Rosenblatt (1928–1971) developed the perceptron, inspired by the functioning of biological neurons. The perceptron is an artificial neural network (ANN) consisting of a single layer of logical units and was one of the first attempts to create a system capable of learning autonomously from data. It can be considered the first machine capable of learning through trial and error, recognizing patterns, and making predictions [6]. At the same time, different pioneer computer scientists began to understand that the functioning of AI was not just the effect of a process of neurons but could be developed through calculations (algorithms) with paths of self-learning based on experience (training). Thus, in 1959, Arthur Lee Samuel (1901–1990) popularized the term "machine learning" (ML) to describe his checkers learning program [7]. The synonym "self-teaching computers" was also used in this period. At the same time, several advancements in computer science were reached and other programs to play checkers and chess were designed, in the 1960s.

After these enthusiastic initial steps, in the 1970s, AI faced several challenges that slowed its progress, leading to a period known as the "AI winter" [8]. Technical limits were underscored, leading to skepticism about the future of neural networks. For example, researchers demonstrated the limitations of perceptrons in solving complex problems. Furthermore, the low returns on investment raised questions about the effectiveness of this technology [5]. Subsequently, the 1980s witnessed a significant resurgence in AI research and development, driven mainly by symbolic AI. Expert Systems and knowledge-based systems were developed as tools to solve complex problems by leveraging extensive knowledge bases represented primarily as if-then rules. For example, AI programs featuring interaction with the world through natural language were developed [9]. Other key steps were reached. The Stanford Cart, a TV-equipped mobile robot, was capable of performing complex physical tasks, such as navigating an environment with obstacles while transporting objects [10]. This demonstrated the potential for robots to manipulate physical objects autonomously, opening new perspectives for practical AI applications.

A paramount step was the development, in 1986, of the backpropagation algorithm, by Geoffrey Hinton. This algorithm, which leverages error feedback in learning processes, significantly improved the ability of neural networks to adapt to data and learn [11]. Significantly, backpropagation addressed the problem of the representation of hierarchy and allowed relationships to be distinguished at different levels.

Despite these notable advancements, toward the end of the 1980s and early 1990s, AI faced new challenges and another winter season [5]. Expert systems showed several limitations, including dependency on initially provided information and limited adaptability across domains. Additionally, maintaining and updating the knowledge base required significant efforts and costs, leading to reduced investment in AI research, which at the time was still heavily reliant on government funding.

Nevertheless, the late 1990s and early 2000s marked the beginning of a new era for AI, driven by advancements in ML and the emergence of big data as well as the start of considerable private research and investments. In 1997, IBM's Deep Blue program obtained an unexpected victory over chess grandmaster Garry Kasparov. In these years, different ML algorithms were made available for classification and regression tasks, providing solutions for a wide range of applications, from image recognition to bioinformatics. Consequently, AI has experienced remarkable progress fueled by the explosion of ML and deep learning (DL) networks.

In the 2010s, the introduction of DL neural networks, such as AlexNet, marked a turning point for AI. These models, capable of learning complex representations from data, revolutionized many fields, including natural language processing and computer vision [12]. Simultaneously, significant progress in hardware technology, particularly the development of high-performance graphics processing units (GPUs), provided the necessary computational power for training complex models. In 2017, the Libratus program, developed by Carnegie Mellon University, triumphed in the "brains vs. artificial intelligence: Upping the Ante" poker tournament.

Additionally, the sharing of open-source frameworks like TensorFlow and PyTorch, supported by major tech companies, allowed access to advanced AI tools, enabling researchers and developers to experiment, innovate, and collaborate more effectively. More importantly, as every AI system requires training on data, the 2010s also ushered in the era of big data, characterized by the exponential growth of data from various sources, including smartphones, social media, IoT devices, and enterprise systems [5]. The volume, variety, and velocity of data are opening unprecedented opportunities for AI development [13]. The immense value of big data is now undeniable and numerous prominent global corporations, including Facebook, Google, Amazon, Apple, and Microsoft have been actively investing in AI research and integrating innovative developments into their commercial operations.

2.2 Definition and Subtypes of Artificial Intelligence

From the Dartmouth Conference, in 1956, several definitions of AI have been proposed to better characterize this discipline. It is assumed that AI can be defined as a technology that enables computers and machines to simulate human intelligence and problem-solving capabilities. Consequently, task-based definitions have been proposed to further explain the skills and tasks associated with AI. For example, computer scientist Nils John Nilsson describes AI as a technology that "functions appropriately and with foresight in its environment" [14]. Others emphasize AI's ability to perceive, pursue goals, initiate actions, and learn from feedback loops [15]. Similarly, the High-Level Expert Group on Artificial Intelligence (AI HLEG) of the European Commission (EC) defines AI as "systems that display intelligent behavior by analyzing their environment and taking actions—with some degree of autonomy—to achieve specific goals" [16]. Regardless of the different definitions, key concepts of AI are the possibility of implementing technologies to allow "machines" to develop typical properties of the human mind, such as learning, reasoning, problem-solving, perception, language understanding, and decision-making: simply, AI systems mimic humans' cognitive functions.

Significantly, since the term AI refers to a multifaceted field, the classification of different AI approaches is challenging. A commonly adopted classification modality distinguishes AI into artificial narrow intelligence (ANI), artificial general intelligence (AGI), and artificial super intelligence (ASI), each with its characteristics, practical uses, applications, and limitations. What distinguishes them from each other is their ability to emulate human characteristics and the technologies they employ to do so. Also known as weak AI, ANI is specialized in a specific task or limited activity [8]. This type of AI is designed to perform specific tasks efficiently but cannot understand or tackle tasks beyond its domain of expertise. ANIs are commonly used across various applications such as speech recognition, image recognition, recommendation systems, algorithmic trading, search engines, and many other fields. These systems are designed to automate specific tasks and enhance efficiency in sectors where machines can surpass human capabilities in terms of speed or precision. However, ANI cannot autonomously adapt to tasks outside of its designed scope or develop new skills or competencies. Also indicated as strong AI, AGI represents the evolutionary phase of AI where machines will have the capability to think and make decisions much like humans. The goal of AGI is to create machines capable of performing multifunctional tasks and acting as realistic and equally intelligent assistants to humans in everyday life. Briefly, weak AI is specialized and task-specific, while strong AI aims to replicate human-like intelligence across a wide range of activities and contexts. Finally, ASI is the stage of AI where computer capabilities will surpass those of humans. It is a theoretical concept referring to a highly advanced form of AI superior to human cognitive abilities. ASI remains a distant prospect at present, representing an advanced and hypothetical phase of AI development, built upon technologies such as supercomputers, and quantum hardware.

A coarse but effective distinction in AI pertains to its purpose, dividing it into predictive AI and generative AI. Predictive AI focuses on forecasting future events or outcomes based on historical data. It involves algorithms that analyze patterns and trends to make informed predictions, such as diagnosing diseases, or forecasting outcomes. Some types of AI, such as those with advanced integrated neurological functions like vision, possess specific analytical properties. Computer vision (CV) is another field of AI that enables computers to interpret and understand visual information from the world, much like human vision. It involves the development of algorithms and systems that can analyze, process, and make decisions based on images or video data. Key applications of CV include image classification, object detection, facial recognition, image segmentation, and scene understanding. Notably, CV itself is not inherently predictive AI, but it can incorporate predictive elements depending on its application. For example, in emotional analysis, CV can predict emotional states based on facial expressions. On the other hand, generative AI is designed to create new content or data that resembles existing data. This includes generating text, images, music, or even entire virtual environments. The distinction is particularly relevant given the remarkable development of generative AI, especially with the release of Large Language Models (LLMs) that can generate coherent and contextually relevant text, or other types of output, based on input prompts. LLMs are natural language processing (NLP) developments. More properly, NLP is a specialized field of AI focused on understanding and manipulating human language. In the medical domain, NLP is instrumental in computerized clinical decision support systems, healthcare management improvements through feedback analysis, and tele-triage services via chatbots. In pain management, NLP can summarize clinical notes and develop dialogue systems for patient interaction and support. It can also aid in creating question-answering systems to provide accurate pain management information. In pain research, NLP extracts information from text-based sources like electronic medical records and patient-reported outcomes, offering a comprehensive understanding of the patient's pain experience and identifying patterns or trends in pain management.

In the context of this chapter, ML and DL will be distinctly highlighted to facilitate a clear and thorough exploration. ML involves algorithms designed to make decisions and predictions based on data analysis. It empowers systems to learn and improve from experience without explicit programming. On the other hand, DL employs artificial neural networks (ANNs) composed of multiple layers of interconnected nodes inspired by the human brain. DL excels in learning intricate representations of data through hierarchical abstraction. For example, LLMs and CV technologies are based on DL architectures [17].

2.3 Machine Learning

2.3.1 ML Subtypes

ML can be broadly categorized into several types, each serving different purposes. A basic distinction divides ML into supervised, unsupervised, and reinforcement learning processes. Supervised learning involves training a model on labeled data, where inputs are paired with corresponding outputs (from the known input to the known predicted output) [18]. For example, predicting the occurrence of a disease based on features like symptoms and diagnostic findings using historical data with known clinical presentations and outcomes. Unsupervised learning, on the other hand, deals with unlabeled data to find hidden patterns or structures, such as clustering customer segments based on clinical behaviors without predefined labels (from the known input to the unknown output). Reinforcement learning focuses on training an agent to make decisions by interacting with an environment and learning from rewards or penalties. For instance, teaching a robot to navigate a maze where it learns to avoid obstacles and reach the goal through trial and error. Researchers often include semi-supervised processes among the ML subtypes. Semi-supervised learning combines both labeled and unlabeled data to improve learning accuracy; it is useful when labeled data is limited.

The ML models perform classification or regression tasks: classification identifies or categorizes an element such as a disease, whereas regression is used to produce a numerical output as a quantitative evaluation, for example, a score. The type of task analysis depends on the algorithm implemented.

2.3.2 Algorithms

ML employs algorithms as operative instruments. The term "algorithm" is derived from the name of the ninth-century Persian mathematician Mohammed ibn Musa al-Kharizmi. An algorithm is a well-defined sequence of instructions or rules designed to solve a specific problem or perform a particular task. It serves as a step-by-step procedure that outlines precisely what actions to take in various scenarios to achieve a desired outcome. Concerning the general functioning, an algorithm requires clearly defined steps, inputs, and outputs, and must always terminate after a finite number of steps. These steps can involve operations like arithmetic calculations, data comparisons, logical operations, and more. In computer programming, algorithms are implemented in various languages and frameworks.

Available ML algorithms vary in complexity and application. For instance, linear regression is a basic algorithm for predicting continuous outputs, fitting a linear equation to data points. Decision trees construct tree-like structures to organize data based on decision rules at each node by using a series of explicit if-then rules on features. This algorithm is useful for tasks like customer churn prediction. Random forest (RF) is included among the same family of algorithms. Each tree in the RF is built from the random sample of the data. If we consider a decision tree as an individual, then a forest would be a collection of people with varying viewpoints. When a significant number of people hold the same opinion, it is probably correct. This concept underlies the RF approach. Thus, a decision tree is a single predictive model that splits data into branches based on feature values to make decisions. In contrast, an RF combines multiple decision trees, each trained on different subsets of the data, to improve accuracy and robustness. Support vector machine (SVM) is another most implemented algorithm. It finds optimal hyperplanes (i.e., boundaries that separate different classes of data points in a multi-dimensional space) to separate data into different classes, employed in image classification tasks like distinguishing cats from dogs. The relevance vector machine (RVM) classification technique is a Bayesian extension of the SVM algorithm. RVM typically results in a much sparser model compared to SVM. This sparsity is achieved by identifying and retaining only the most relevant data points, known as relevance vectors, rather than relying on a large subset of the training data as SVM does with support vectors. The reduction in the number of relevance vectors leads to more efficient computation and can improve the interpretability of the model, as it focuses on the most influential data points driving the classification decisions. Additionally, gradient boosting (XGBoost) builds a model in a stage-wise fashion from weak learners, typically decision trees. Each new tree is fit on the negative gradient of the loss function of the prediction of the ensemble so far. This algorithm has a built-in mechanism to handle missing data, which makes it robust in real-world scenarios where data can be incomplete. Moreover, XGBoost implements tree pruning (pruning of split points that do not contribute significantly) and regularization (lasso and ridge regularization to penalize complex models) to control overfitting (i.e., the model learns the training data too well, capturing noise and details that do not generalize to new, unseen data). It is widely used for classification and regression tasks due to its speed, regularization capabilities, and ability to handle large datasets.

Interpolation methods are mathematical techniques used to estimate unknown values that fall within the range of known data points. They are commonly employed in various fields such as data analysis, computer graphics, and engineering to create smooth curves or surfaces from discrete data. Some machine learning algorithms can be considered interpolative, particularly when they focus on fitting data points closely. For example, k-nearest neighbors (k-NN) can be seen as a form of interpolation because it predicts the label or value of a new data point based on the labels or values of its nearest neighbors in the training set.

The foundation of reinforcement learning is built on the concept of a Markov decision process (MDP). It is a mathematical framework used to model decision-making in environments where outcomes are partly random and partly under the control of a decision-maker. In an MDP, the primary objective is to optimize the policy, or strategy, that the agent follows to maximize the cumulative reward over time. This involves not just considering immediate rewards but also anticipating the long-term consequences of actions, thereby ensuring that the overall future cumulative reward is as high as possible. Although MDP is not an algorithm, different algorithms such as value iteration and policy iteration are used to solve MDPs by finding the optimal policy that maximizes the cumulative reward.

In an ML process, different algorithms are usually tested, structuring various models, and their performances are evaluated. A summary of ML algorithms is presented in Table 2.1.

Classification predicts the categorical class labels of new observations based on past observations with known labels. It involves identifying which category an object belongs given its features. Regression is used to predict continuous outcomes. It models the relationship between dependent variables (features) and independent variables (outcome) in the form of a mathematical function.

2.3.3 ML Modeling

Every ML journey begins with defining the task and culminates in deploying the model. Connecting these endpoints reveals several identifiable steps. However, the system is not static; it evolves dynamically throughout its stages, adapting to address emerging issues. High-performance standards and rigorous quality controls are essential throughout the process. Therefore, the role of the analyst is prominent for the final result.

Table 2.1 Main algorithms for machine learning and applications in medicine

Algorithm	Explanation	Applications in medicine
Linear regression	Finds the linear relationship between dependent and independent variables	Predicting disease progression based on patient data
Logistic regression	Used for binary classification tasks, estimating the probability of a binary outcome	Diagnosing diseases based on symptoms and risk factors
Decision trees	Hierarchical tree-like structures used for classification and regression tasks	Predicting patient outcomes based on medical history
Random forest	Ensemble learning method using multiple decision trees to improve accuracy and robustness	Identifying high-risk patients for proactive care
Support vector machines	Classifies data by finding the hyperplane that best separates different classes	Image recognition in radiology for tumor detection
Relevance vector machine	For regression and classification tasks. It provides probabilistic predictions (Bayesian inference to determine the relevance of each data point) giving not just a point estimate but also a measure of uncertainty	Signal processing (noise reduction and signal reconstruction). Medical diagnosis where understanding the uncertainty of predictions is crucial
Gradient boosting	It builds models sequentially and can iteratively improve predictions by focusing on the errors made by previous models	Disease diagnosis, prognosis and outcome prediction, medical imaging
K-nearest neighbors	Classifies data based on similarity to neighboring data points	Identifying similar patient cases for treatment planning
Naive Bayes	Probabilistic classifier based on Bayes' theorem with strong independence assumptions	Predicting the likelihood of diseases from symptoms
Neural networks	Deep learning models inspired by biological neural networks, capable of learning complex patterns	Analyzing genetic data for personalized medicine

The process of applying ML involves several steps: *data collection* and *preprocessing* to ensure data quality, *explorative data analysis*, feature selection or extraction to represent data effectively, *model selection* and *training* using appropriate algorithms, *evaluation* of validation data to assess performance, and finally deployment into production environments for real-time decision-making [8].

Data collection and preprocessing are key steps. They must ensure data quality by cleaning, transforming, and normalizing it for training. Given that outputs hinge directly on the provided data and AI predictions can significantly impact clinical decisions, precise structuring and manipulation of the preprocessing dataset are paramount. During this pivotal stage, clinicians must collaborate closely with computer scientists to ensure models are not only mathematically optimal but also aligned with the specific clinical contexts they are intended to serve.

Exploratory data analysis (EDA) serves the critical purpose of uncovering trends and patterns within datasets, constituting a dynamic link to preceding data preprocessing stages. Data scientists leverage EDA to meticulously examine datasets, summarizing key characteristics often through data visualization techniques. This approach aids in identifying the optimal data manipulation strategies, facilitating pattern detection, anomaly identification, and hypothesis testing across one or multiple hypotheses. Essentially, EDA delves beyond formal modeling and hypothesis testing, offering a deeper insight into dataset variables and their intricate relationships. Moreover, it validates the appropriateness of statistical techniques applied in data analysis. In other words, EDA has a pivotal impact on the performance of ML models. Thorough EDA helps in selecting appropriate modeling techniques, tuning hyperparameters effectively, and assessing model assumptions. It mitigates the risk of overfitting or underfitting models by ensuring that the chosen algorithms are well-suited to the data characteristics revealed during EDA. Practically, EDA involves statistical summaries and visual methods such as histograms, scatter plots, and other graphical tools to analyze features comprehensively. Depending on the research goals, EDA encompasses univariate nongraphical analysis, suitable for examining a single variable, univariate graphical analysis, which includes tools like stem-and-leaf plots, histograms, and box plots, multivariate nongraphical analysis, utilized to explore relationships between two or more variables through cross-tabulation or statistical methods, and multivariate graphical analysis, employing visualizations such as bar charts, scatter plots, bubble charts, and heat maps to illustrate connections between datasets. Libraries for data analysis and visualization such as Python libraries Pandas for data manipulation, and Seaborn and Matplotlib for generating plots, are commonly used. Automated EDA tools are available, such as AutoEDA by XanderHorn [17].

The model building is a dynamic process. The training and evaluation stages include several steps aimed at developing a predictive model that generalizes well to unseen data. Initially, the training phase begins with the selection of a model architecture and algorithm suited to the problem domain. The analyst's role is once again of paramount importance. For example, in a decision tree, different parameters are used to control the complexity of the tree such as *max_depth, max_leaf_nodes, min_samples_leaf.* Moreover, in a Bayesian approach, the relationship between features requires human engagement. Yet, in the RF classifier, the number of trees and the number of features (hyperparameters) must be accurately chosen. Using training data, the model learns to adjust its parameters iteratively to minimize the difference between predicted outcomes and actual values, typically guided by an objective function like mean squared error or cross-entropy loss. Sophisticated training strategies can be also adopted. Curriculum learning, for instance, leverages the concept of structured learning progression, resulting in more robust and efficient ML models. In this process, data is organized in a meaningful order, typically starting with easier examples and gradually progressing to more difficult ones. This approach mimics the way humans learn, beginning with simple concepts and building up to more complex ones. In Transfer Learning, models are pre-trained on a large dataset and subsequently fine-tuned on a smaller, task-specific dataset. Additionally, thanks to efficient algorithms that can update models quickly, Online Learning models are trained incrementally as new data becomes available, rather than in one batch.

Once trained, the model's performance is evaluated using a separate validation dataset to assess its ability to generalize beyond the training data. Therefore, model training involves selecting an appropriate algorithm, optimizing parameters, and evaluating performance on validation datasets using metrics for classification and regression tasks.

The notion of accuracy is crucial for assessing performance of classification models. To illustrate it, a binary classification task, such as positive vs. negative could be considered. Given a test set consisting of N instances, true positives (TP) are the number of positive instances correctly identified, and true negatives (TN) are the number of negative instances correctly identified. It can be expressed as a percentage. Accuracy is then calculated:

$$\text{ACC\%} = \frac{\text{TP} + \text{TN}}{N\,\text{samples}} \cdot 100$$

Consequently, higher values indicate better performance.

Recall and precision are other key metrics. In binary problems, Recall is also known as the true positive rate and corresponds to sensitivity, while the true negative rate is referred to as specificity. For multi-class problems, accuracy is determined by considering the TP for each class, and recall and precision can be calculated for each class individually.

Taken together, evaluation metrics such as accuracy, precision, recall, and F1-score provide quantitative measures of the model's predictive accuracy and robustness (Table 2.2).

Other metrics are used for regression tasks. They include, for instance, the mean squared error (MSE) which represents the average squared differences between predicted and actual values, the root mean squared error (RMSE), the Log Loss (Logarithmic Loss) which indicates the measure of the performance of a classification model whose output is a probability value, the Matthews Correlation Coefficient

Table 2.2 Key metrics for classification tasks

Metric	Description	Formula	Use case
Accuracy	The proportion of correctly predicted instances out of the total instances	$\frac{\text{TP}+\text{TN}}{N\,\text{samples}}$	Overall performance of classification models
Precision	The proportion of true positive predictions out of all positive predictions made by the model	$\frac{\text{TP}}{\text{TP}+\text{FP}}$	Evaluates the model's accuracy in positive predictions
Recall (sensitivity)	The proportion of true positives detected by the model out of all actual positives	$\frac{\text{TP}}{\text{TP}+\text{FN}}$	Measures the model's ability to identify all positive cases
F1 score	The harmonic mean of precision and recall	$2 \cdot \frac{\text{Precision} \cdot \text{Recall}}{\text{Precision} + \text{Recall}}$	
Specificity	The proportion of true negatives correctly identified out of all actual negatives	$\frac{\text{TN}}{\text{TN}+\text{FP}}$	Measures the model's ability to identify all negative cases

(MCC), illustrating the quality of binary classifications, considering true and false positives and negatives, and other parameters. Additionally, mean absolute error (MAE) is a metric used to evaluate the accuracy of a model in regression tasks. It measures the average magnitude of the errors between predicted values and the actual values. Lower MAE values indicate better predictive accuracy; therefore, it is intuitive that an MAE of zero indicates perfect accuracy (ACC = 1), where all predicted values exactly match the actual value. While MAE is less sensitive to outliers compared to MSE because it does not square the errors, it gives a sense of the average magnitude of the errors in a set of predictions, which is easy to understand and interpret.

A key metric is the area under the curve—receiver operating characteristic (AUC-ROC). The ROC curve is a graphical representation that plots the true positive rate against the false positive rate across different threshold settings. The AUC measures the area under this curve, providing an aggregate performance metric across all possible classification thresholds. AUC values range from 0 to 1, where a value closer to 1 indicates a model with excellent discriminative ability, meaning it is better at distinguishing between positive and negative cases (Fig. 2.1).

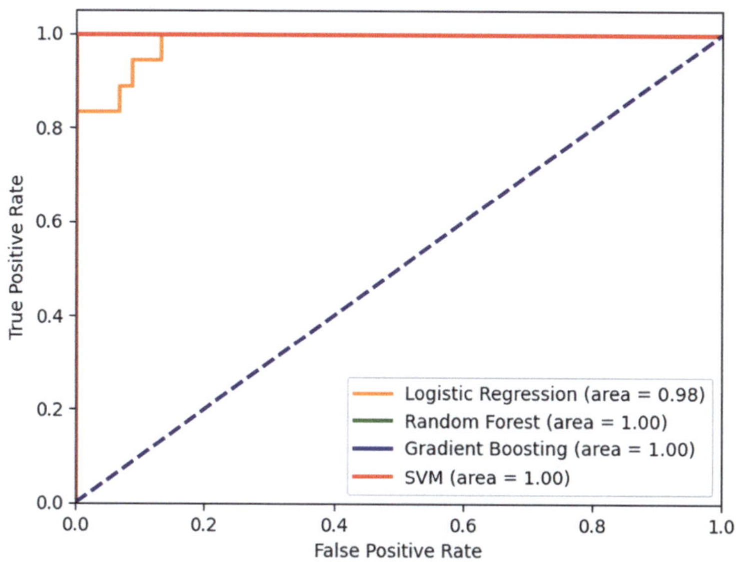

Fig. 2.1 The receiver operating characteristic (ROC) curve provides an important and immediate visual impact, offering a clear and intuitive representation of a model's performance across different classification thresholds. In this example, four machine learning algorithms are evaluated. A classifier whose ROC curve falls on the diagonal (blue dashed) is essentially making random predictions. For every positive instance, it has a 50% chance of predicting it as positive and a 50% chance of predicting it as negative, and similarly for negative instances. Therefore, the true positive rate (sensitivity) is equal to the false positive rate, meaning the classifier's predictions are no better than chance. Considering the area under the curve (AUC), the area under the diagonal line is 0.5, which corresponds to the AUC of a random classifier. AUC values range from 0 to 1, with values above 0.5 indicating better than random performance

Table 2.3 Confusion matrix format

	Predicted positive	Predicted negative
Actual positive	True positive (TP)	False negative (FN)
Actual negative	False positive (FP)	True negative (TN)

Also termed as concordance statistic or *C*-index, *C*-statistic is a measure of goodness of fit for binary outcomes in a logistic regression model. Briefly, it is similar to the AUR ROC and ranges from 0 to 1.

As previously introduced, for classification metrics, actual and predicted values are related. The relationship occurs within the confusion matrix. The confusion matrix is a powerful tool for evaluating the performance of classification algorithms and provides a detailed breakdown of how the model's predictions compare to the actual outcomes. It can be used for binary (e.g., disease vs. no disease) or multi-class classification. A confusion matrix for a binary classification problem typically has the following format (Table 2.3):

From the matrix, it emerges that two "diagonals" are established: one for true predictions (true positive and true negative) and one for false ones (false positive and false negative).

During evaluation, the overfitting and underfitting phenomena must be addressed. Overfitting occurs when a model learns to capture noise or irrelevant patterns from the training data, leading to poor performance on new (unseen) data. This can be detected if the model performs exceptionally well on training data but poorly on validation or test data. As illustrated in Fig. 2.1, the models tested exhibit exceptional performance, with accuracy approaching perfection. However, this level of performance also indicates that the models may have been excessively trained or overfitted to the specific dataset used for training and testing. As a result, while the models perform extraordinarily well on the data they were trained and validated on, their ability to generalize to other datasets or real-world scenarios may be compromised. This can lead to overly optimistic performance metrics that do not accurately reflect the model's effectiveness in practical applications.

Different techniques can be used to mitigate overfitting. For example, regularization methods like L1/L2 regularization, dropout, and early stopping prevent the model from becoming too complex or too specialized for the training data. On the other hand, underfitting arises when a model is too simplistic to capture the underlying patterns in the data, resulting in poor performance on both training and validation sets. This issue is typically addressed by using more complex models, increasing the number of training epochs, or enhancing feature representation through feature engineering.

At this stage, the model can be applied in real-world scenarios. Continuous monitoring to maintain performance and identify degradation requiring retraining is required [19].

2.4 Deep Learning

Unlike traditional ML approaches that rely on explicit feature extraction and selection, DL models automatically learn hierarchical representations of data through multiple layers of interconnected elements. These networks are organized hierarchically, with each layer processing increasingly abstract features extracted from the data [20]. Briefly, artificial neural architectures (ANNs) are composed of artificial neurons, known as units or nodes, organized into layers. These layers together form the structure of the network. Depending on the complexity of the task, a layer may contain anywhere from a few dozen to millions of units. Typically, an ANN includes an input layer, one or more hidden layers, and an output layer that generates the final response based on the processed data. ANNs are inspired by the structure and operations of biological neurons. The input layer receives signals from external sources such as a dataset, which it then passes to the hidden layer, the second layer. In the hidden layer, each neuron processes the inputs from the previous layer by computing a weighted sum and transmitting the result to neurons in the subsequent layer. These connections, or weights, adjust during the training process to optimize the model's performance. Bias is an additional parameter in each neuron that helps the activation function—a mathematical function applied to the weighted sum of inputs to introduce non-linearity—shift to fit the data better. In other words, functionally, the weights correspond to the biological synapses where the strength of these connections affects signal transmission (Fig. 2.2).

Given these properties, DL models excel in tasks such as image and speech recognition, natural language understanding, and medical diagnosis due to their ability to automatically learn intricate patterns and representations from raw data. However, they also require careful tuning of hyperparameters, regularization techniques, and extensive data preprocessing to avoid issues like overfitting and ensure robust performance.

There are several types of DL architectures, each tailored to different types of data and tasks. Convolutional neural networks (CNNs), for instance, are particularly effective for image and video recognition tasks by leveraging spatial hierarchies. These architectures have revolutionized the field of CV. Yet, recurrent neural networks (RNNs) are designed to handle sequential data and are widely used in NLP and time-series analysis. Long short-term memory networks (LSTMs), a variant of RNNs, address the vanishing gradient problem and are capable of learning long-term dependencies in sequential data [21]. The main ANN architectures and applications in medicine are summarized in Table 2.4.

Architectures vary in complexity, with the potential to incorporate elements that play significant functional roles. For instance, LLMs are developed using the transformer architectures. These neural network models utilize self-attention mechanisms, allowing the model to consider the entire context of the input rather than being limited to fixed-size windows. They also employ multi-head attention to capture complex contextual relationships within input sequences. Key components of the transformer architecture include encoder and decoder structures, which respectively handle the processing of input sequences and the generation of output

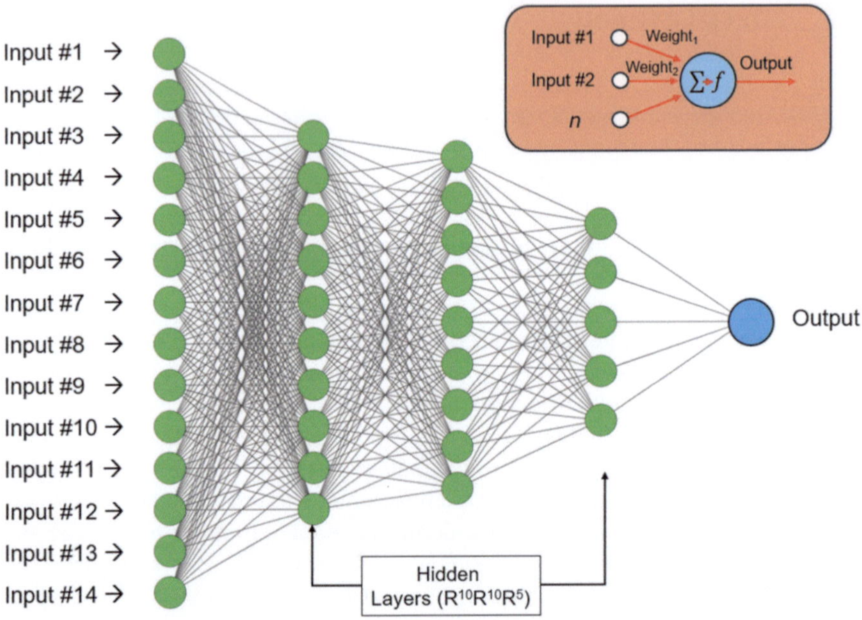

Fig. 2.2 Scheme of a simple artificial neural architecture. The input layer ($R = 14$) receives data from the external environment (dataset), which the network needs to process. Since the primary function of the input layer is to pass the input data into the network without any processing, this data passes through three hidden layers, where it is transformed into information that the output layer can use. Each connection is assigned a weight that influences how the data is transferred between units and represents the strength and direction (positive or negative) of the influence one neuron has on another. Each node in a hidden layer receives inputs from all nodes in the previous layer, applies a set of weights, adds a bias, and passes the result through an activation function (e.g., sigmoid, ReLU) to produce an output. Weights determine the importance of each input in the computation; therefore, a higher weight means a stronger influence. The weighted inputs are summed, and the result is passed through an activation function ($\sum \cdot f$) to introduce non-linearity and enable the network to learn complex patterns. As data moves through these connections, the network learns and refines its understanding, ultimately producing an output in response to the initial input. During training, the weights are updated iteratively to minimize the error in the network's predictions. For each iteration, the model calculates the gradient of the error for each weight and adjusts the weights in the direction that reduces the error. The nature of the output layer depends on the specific task (e.g., binary classification, multi-class classification, regression)

sequences [22]. Furthermore, generative architectures, particularly those used in generating data such as images, text, or audio, have a specific structure designed to produce new, realistic samples. Examples of generative architectures are generative adversarial networks (GANs) and variational autoencoders (VAEs). The former is composed of a generator and a discriminator. The generator creates new data samples from random noise, while the discriminator evaluates whether these samples are real or fake, effectively training the generator to produce increasingly realistic data. On the other hand, VAEs consist of an encoder and a decoder. The encoder compresses the input data into a latent space representation, and the decoder reconstructs the data from this representation, enabling the generation of new samples by

Table 2.4 Deep learning architectures in medicine. In deep networks, especially those with many layers or over long sequences, gradients can diminish significantly as they are backpropagated from the output layer back to the input layer. This phenomenon can hinder the ability of the network to learn effectively because small gradients lead to minimal updates to the weights and biases of the network, slowing down or even halting learning altogether. Abbreviations: NLP, natural language processing; HER, Electronic health record

Architecture	Explanation	Applications in medicine	Key algorithms
Convolutional neural networks (CNNs)	Designed for processing grid-like data, extracting hierarchical features through convolutional layers	Medical imaging (e.g., MRI segmentation, X-ray abnormality detection, histopathology classification)	AlexNet, VGGNet, ResNet, Inception
Recurrent neural networks (RNNs)	Process sequential data while maintaining the memory of previous inputs (tasks with temporal dependencies)	Time-series analysis (e.g., patient outcome prediction, disease progression modeling, physiological signal monitoring)	Vanilla RNN, gated recurrent unit (GRU)
Long short-term memory networks (LSTMs)	Type of RNN for addressing the vanishing gradient problem. It is effective in capturing long-term dependencies in sequential data	EHR analysis (e.g., readmission prediction, medication adherence modeling, patient trajectory)	LSTM, BiLSTM (Bidirectional LSTM)
Generative adversarial networks (GANs)	Consists of generator and discriminator networks trained adversarially to generate synthetic data resembling real data	Synthetic data generation (e.g., medical image synthesis, rare disease simulation, dataset augmentation)	DCGAN (Deep Convolutional GAN), CycleGAN
Transformers	Attention-based models originally for NLP tasks, adept at capturing context from large amounts of sequential data	Clinical language processing (e.g., clinical note understanding, medical literature summarization, translation)	BERT, GPT, T5, Transformer-XL

sampling from the latent space. Both architectures are pivotal in various applications, from image synthesis to data augmentation and beyond [23–25]. Recently, different multimodal LLMs have been developed. Since in these models, input and output can be both multimodal, they can generate content across a spectrum of formats including text, images, audio, and video.

The functioning of DL models involves activation, training, and inference. In biological neurons, activation refers to the neuron's firing rate when the received impulses are strong enough to surpass a threshold. In artificial units, activation is performed by an activation function, a mathematical function that maps the input to the output and determines whether a neuron should fire. During the training phase, the model learns from a large amount of labeled data, adjusting its parameters—weights and biases—iteratively to minimize the difference between predicted and actual outputs. Weights are the parameters within the network that transform input data within the neurons, while biases are additional parameters that allow the activation function to be shifted to the left or right, which can help the model better fit the data. This learning process typically involves an algorithm called backpropagation, where the error is propagated backward through the network to update weights and biases. This learning process adjusts the weights between nodes based on the error between predicted and actual outcomes. Optimization algorithms such as stochastic gradient descent (SGD), adaptive moment estimation (Adam), and root mean square propagation (RMSprop) are used to adjust these weights and biases efficiently.

Notably, training these models often requires significant computational resources, especially for large-scale datasets and complex architectures. High-performance computing environments with GPUs or tensor processing units (TPUs) are typically used to accelerate the training process. In contrast, during the inference phase, the trained model makes predictions on new, unseen data. This phase is less computationally intensive than training, as it involves a forward pass through the network where the input data is transformed through the learned weights and biases to generate an output.

One of the challenges with DL models is their inherent complexity, often leading to their characterization as "black boxes" [26]. This term refers to the difficulty in interpreting and understanding the inner workings of these models, underscoring that their decision-making processes are not easily transparent. This serious lack of interpretability can be particularly concerning in critical applications such as medicine, where understanding the rationale behind predictions is essential for trust and accountability. To address this issue, the field of explainable AI (XAI) has emerged. It focuses on developing techniques that make AI models more interpretable and transparent without significantly compromising their performance. XAI fosters safety and trust by clarifying the "how" and "why" behind automated decision-making across a range of applications, including bio-inspired systems, virtual agents, emotion and affective analysis, robotics, and medical diagnostics. Different XAI approaches, such as attention mechanisms, saliency maps, and model-agnostic methods like Local Interpretable Model-agnostic Explanations (LIME) and SHapley Additive exPlanations (SHAP), are employed to shed light on how DL models arrive at their decisions, thereby increasing their usability and trustworthiness in sensitive and high-stakes domains [27].

2.5 Ethical Considerations

The integration of AI into medicine and healthcare raises several ethical and practical considerations. A crucial aspect is the autonomy of technology and the possibility that it might "escape" human control, combined with the low reliability of its results and the production of biased outcomes. Many efforts are being made in this direction and human-in-the-loop (HITL) and algorithmic stewardship principles are being structured [28]. The concept of HITL refers to a design approach in AI where human judgment and decision-making are integrated into the AI system's processes. In other words, according to a hybrid human-machine model, to ensure that AI systems remain aligned with human values and ethical standards, researchers interact with and oversee AI algorithms, providing feedback and making final decisions when necessary [29]. Furthermore, algorithmic stewardship involves the responsible design, development, deployment, and monitoring of AI and algorithmic systems. HITL and algorithm stewardship are algorethics processes, a new field of study that, according to Benanti "focuses on issues such as transparency and accountability of algorithms, data bias, and accountability." The goal of AI ethics or machine ethics is to ensure thorough and collaborative oversight of the processes that shape the interactions between technology, society, and individuals [30, 31].

One major concern is data privacy and security. AI systems rely on large amounts of patient data to function effectively, and ensuring the confidentiality and security of this data is paramount. Healthcare providers must adhere to strict data protection regulations and implement robust cybersecurity measures to prevent data breaches. Importantly, since AI systems are fed by data health information exchange (HIE) pathways should be implemented to prevent the risk of data monopolies. In the United States, healthcare organizations must comply with the Health Insurance Portability and Accountability Act (HIPAA) to ensure the privacy and security of patient information. HIPAA establishes standards for data security in healthcare and mandates the protection of electronic health information, requiring organizations to implement measures to prevent unauthorized access [32].

Data bias is another significant issue. Significantly, since ML and DL approaches are data-driven, they are strictly conditioned to the available data. AI systems, for instance, can inadvertently perpetuate existing biases present in the data they are trained on, leading to unequal treatment outcomes. For instance, if an AI system is trained on data that predominantly represents a particular demographic, it may not perform as well for other populations. Ensuring diversity in training datasets and implementing fairness checks are essential steps in mitigating this risk [33].

Before adopting an AI-based technology in clinical practice, it must undergo rigorous validation to ensure its accuracy and reliability. Clinical trials and real-world testing are necessary to evaluate the performance of AI systems in diverse patient populations and clinical settings. Additionally, integrating AI into existing clinical workflows requires careful planning and training to ensure seamless adoption without disrupting patient care [34].

Given the enormous concerns associated with the use of AI, regulatory policy interventions are mandatory. In June 2024, the European Parliament and Council approved the Artificial Intelligence Act. This regulation aims to protect fundamental rights, democracy, the rule of law, and environmental sustainability from high-risk AI while fostering innovation and establishing Europe's leadership in AI. It introduces obligations based on AI's risk levels and bans applications threatening citizens' rights, such as biometric categorization, untargeted facial image scraping, emotion recognition in sensitive environments, social scoring, and certain predictive policing methods. The use of biometric identification systems by law enforcement is generally prohibited, with narrow exceptions requiring strict safeguards and judicial authorization. High-risk AI applications in critical areas like infrastructure, education, healthcare, and law enforcement must assess risks, maintain transparency, and ensure human oversight. Citizens can submit complaints and receive explanations regarding AI decisions affecting their rights [35]. In late 2023, the President of the United States issued an executive order titled "Safe, Secure, and Trustworthy Development and Use of AI." This comprehensive order addresses various policy areas, establishing new standards for AI safety and security, implementing measures to protect citizens' privacy from AI-related risks, advancing equity and civil rights, supporting workers, promoting innovation and competition, strengthening US leadership on the global stage, and ensuring the responsible and effective government use of AI [36]. The EU and the US collaborate on AI through the Trade and Technology Council (TTC), where they are jointly developing a roadmap for evaluating and measuring trustworthy AI and managing associated risks.

Nevertheless, methods for assessing AI ethics—specifically evaluating whether an AI system meets ethical standards—are often overlooked in the literature [37].

2.6 Implementation Strategies for Clinicians

Implementing AI in clinical practice involves several practical steps, including selecting appropriate AI tools, training staff, and integrating AI systems with existing workflows. Collaboration with AI developers and ongoing evaluation of AI performance is essential to ensure successful integration. For example, accurate data collection is mandatory. The principle of "garbage in, garbage out" (GIGO) is fundamental to understanding how input information affects the results obtained from a system. Originally applied to programming and computer systems, this concept is equally relevant in the context of AI [38]. Clinicians and researchers should consider the potential negative impact of a language model (e.g., a chatbot) trained on biased data to fully understand its possible consequences. As an example, in 2016, the AI chatbot Tay.ai was taken down less than a day after its launch on Twitter (now X) because it began exhibiting racist and sexist behavior [39].

Another crucial step concerns training and education for healthcare providers. Healthcare providers must receive training and education on AI technologies, their applications, and their limitations. Understanding how to interpret AI-generated insights and incorporate them into clinical decision-making is crucial. In this context, continuous professional development will keep providers updated on the latest advancements in AI.

Finally, overcoming barriers to AI adoption in pain medicine such as resistance to change, lack of understanding, and concerns about cost and data security requires clear communication of AI's benefits. Therefore, it is mandatory to develop multiprofessional projects for demonstrating AI efficacy through, for instance, pilot projects [40].

References

1. McCulloch WS, Pitt W. A logical calculus of the ideas immanent in nervous activity. Bull Math Biophys. 1943;5:115–33. https://doi.org/10.1007/BF02478259.
2. Grzybowski A, Pawlikowska-Łagód K, Lambert WC. A history of artificial intelligence. Clin Dermatol. 2024;42(3):221–9. https://doi.org/10.1016/j.clindermatol.2023.12.016.
3. Turing AM. Computing machinery and intelligence. Mind. 1950;54(236):433–60. https://doi.org/10.1093/mind/LIX.236.433.
4. Kirkebøen G. Descartes's Regulae, mathematics, and modern psychology: "the Noblest example of all" in Light of Turing's (1936) On computable numbers. Hist Psychol. 2000;3:299–325. https://doi.org/10.1037/1093-4510.3.4.299.
5. The history of artificial intelligence. https://sitn.hms.harvard.edu/flash/2017/history-artificial-intelligence/. Last retrieved 2 Jul 2024.
6. Block HD. The perceptron: a model for brain functioning. I Rev Mod Phys. 1962;34:123.
7. Weiss EA. Arthur Lee Samuel (1901-90). IEEE Ann Hist Comput. 1992;14(3):55–69. https://doi.org/10.1109/85.150082.
8. Bellini V, Cascella M, Cutugno F, Russo M, Lanza R, Compagnone C, Bignami EG. Understanding basic principles of artificial intelligence: a practical guide for intensivists. Acta Biomed. 2022;93(5):e2022297. https://doi.org/10.23750/abm.v93i5.13626.
9. A brief history of natural language processing. https://www.dataversity.net/a-brief-history-of-natural-language-processing-nlp/. Last retrieved 2 Jul 2024.
10. Moravec HP. The Stanford Cart and the CMU Rover. Proc IEEE. 1983;71:872–84. https://doi.org/10.1109/PROC.1983.12684.
11. Hinton G. Where do features come from? Cogn Sci. 2014;38(6):1078–101. https://doi.org/10.1111/cogs.12049.
12. Krizhevsky A, Sutskever I, Hinton GE. ImageNet classification with deep convolutional neural networks. Adv Neural Inf Proces Syst. 2012;25:1–9.
13. Bellini V, Cascella M, Montomoli J, Bignami E. From big data's 5Vs to clinical practice's 5Ws: enhancing data-driven decision making in healthcare. J Clin Monit Comput. 2023;37(5):1423–5. https://doi.org/10.1007/s10877-023-01007-3.
14. Nilsson N. The quest for artificial intelligence. Cambridge: Cambridge University Press; 2009.
15. DenkWerk. Artificial intelligence in Nederland: Zelf Aan Het Stuur. 2018. https://denkwerk.online/media/1029/artitificial_intelligence_in_nederland_juli_2018.pdf. Last retrieved 9 Jul 2024.
16. The European Commission's high-level expert group on artificial intelligence. https://ec.europa.eu/futurium/en/system/files/ged/ai_hleg_definition_of_ai_18_december_1.pdf. Last retrieved 9 Jul 2024.
17. Cascella M, Semeraro F, Montomoli J, Bellini V, Piazza O, Bignami E. The breakthrough of large language models release for medical applications: 1-year timeline and perspectives. J Med Syst. 2024;48(1):22. https://doi.org/10.1007/s10916-024-02045-3.
18. Staniak M, Biecek P. The landscape of R packages for automated exploratory data analysis. R J. 2019;11(2):347–69.
19. Cho B, Geng E, Arvind V, Valliani AA, Tang JE, Schwartz J, Dominy C, Cho SK, Kim JS. Understanding artificial intelligence and predictive analytics: a clinically focused review of machine learning techniques. JBJS Rev. 2022;10(3). https://doi.org/10.2106/JBJS.RVW.21.00142.
20. Bini SA. Artificial intelligence, machine learning, deep learning, and cognitive computing: what do these terms mean and how will they impact health care? J Arthroplast. 2018;33(8):2358–61. https://doi.org/10.1016/j.arth.2018.02.067.
21. Deep learning architectures. https://developer.ibm.com/articles/cc-machine-learning-deep-learning-architectures/. Last retrieved 2 Jul 2024.

22. Kalyan KS, Rajasekharan A, Sangeetha S. Ammu: a survey of transformer-based biomedical pretrained language models. J Biomed Inform. 2022;126:103982. https://doi.org/10.1016/j.jbi.2021.103982.
23. Cascella M, Scarpati G, Bignami EG, Cuomo A, Vittori A, Di Gennaro P, Crispo A, Coluccia S. Utilizing an artificial intelligence framework (conditional generative adversarial network) to enhance telemedicine strategies for cancer pain management. J Anesth Analg Crit Care. 2023;3(1):19. https://doi.org/10.1186/s44158-023-00104-8.
24. Chen X, Xia Y, Dall'Armellina E, Ravikumar N, Frangi AF. Joint shape/texture representation learning for cardiovascular disease diagnosis from magnetic resonance imaging. Eur Heart J Imaging Methods Pract. 2024;2(1):qyae042. https://doi.org/10.1093/ehjimp/qyae042.
25. Wang R, Bashyam V, Yang Z, Yu F, Tassopoulou V, Chintapalli SS, Skampardoni I, Sreepada LP, Sahoo D, Nikita K, Abdulkadir A, Wen J, Davatzikos C. Applications of generative adversarial networks in neuroimaging and clinical neuroscience. NeuroImage. 2023;269:119898. https://doi.org/10.1016/j.neuroimage.2023.119898.
26. Zednik C. Solving the black box problem: a normative framework for explainable artificial intelligence. Philos Technol. 2021;34:265–88.
27. Räz T, Beisbart C. The importance of understanding deep learning. Erkenn. 2024;89:1823–40. https://doi.org/10.1007/s10670-022-00605-y.
28. Montomoli J, Bitondo MM, Cascella M, Rezoagli E, Romeo L, Bellini V, Semeraro F, Gamberini E, Frontoni E, Agnoletti V, Altini M, Benanti P, Bignami EG. Algor-ethics: charting the ethical path for AI in critical care. J Clin Monit Comput. 2024;38(4):931–9. https://doi.org/10.1007/s10877-024-01157-y.
29. Bignami E, Montomoli J, Bellini V, Cascella M. Uncovering the power of synergy: a hybrid human-machine model for maximizing AI properties and human expertise. Crit Care. 2023;27(1):330. https://doi.org/10.1186/s13054-023-04598-0.
30. Benanti P. The urgency of an algorethics. Discov Artif Intell. 2023;3:11. https://doi.org/10.1007/s44163-023-00056-6.
31. Allen C, Wallach W, Smit I. Why machine ethics? IEEE Intell Syst. 2006;21(4):12–7.
32. Health Insurance Portability and Accountability Act of 1996 (HIPAA). https://www.cdc.gov/phlp/php/resources/health-insurance-portability-and-accountability-act-of-1996-hipaa.html?CDC_AAref_Val=https://www.cdc.gov/phlp/publications/topic/hipaa.html. Last retrieved 23 Jun 2024.
33. Cascella M, Tracey MC, Petrucci E, Bignami EG. Exploring artificial intelligence in anesthesia: a primer on ethics, and clinical applications. Surgeries. 2023;4(2):264–74. https://doi.org/10.3390/surgeries4020027.
34. Cascella M, Laudani A, Scarpati G, Piazza O. Ethical issues in pain and palliation. Curr Opin Anaesthesiol. 2024;37(2):199–204. https://doi.org/10.1097/ACO.0000000000001345.
35. European Parliament. Artificial Intelligence Act. https://ai-act-law.eu/. Last retrieved 20 Jul 2024.
36. The White House. Executive order on the safe secure and trustworthy development and use of artificial intelligence. https://www.whitehouse.gov/briefing-room/presidential-actions/2023/10/30/executive-order-on-the-safe-secure-and-trustworthy-development-and-use-of-artificial-intelligence/. Last retrieved 20 Jul 2024.
37. Huang C, Zhang Z, Mao B, Yao X. An overview of artificial intelligence ethics. IEEE Trans Artif Intell. 2023;4(4):799–819. https://doi.org/10.1109/TAI.2022.3194503.
38. Bellini V, Montomoli J, Bignami E. Poor quality data, privacy, lack of certifications: the lethal triad of new technologies in intensive care. Intensive Care Med. 2021;47(9):1052–3. https://doi.org/10.1007/s00134-021-06473-4.
39. McGregor S. An incident database. Incident number 6. 2016. https://incidentdatabase.ai/cite/6. Last retrieved 29 Jun 2024.
40. Bignami E, Darhour LJ, Bellini V. Artificial intelligence in extended perioperative medicine. Trends Anaesth Crit Care. 2024;57:101376. https://doi.org/10.1016/j.tacc.2024.101376.

Research in Automatic Pain Assessment 3

3.1 Nociception and Pain

According to the definition released by the International Association for the Study of Pain (IASP) in 2020, pain is "An unpleasant sensory and emotional experience associated with, or resembling that associated with, actual or potential tissue damage" [1]. In physiological conditions, pain represents a rapid "alarm" system, to warn the body that a certain stimulus could lead to injuries, potentially even lethal. Acute pain results from the activation of pain receptors (nociceptors) at the site of application of a stimulus that may or may not cause tissue damage. This acute pain in response to an insult, such as trauma pain or postoperative pain, is a physiological phenomenon but may be associated with significant physical, psychological, and emotional distress. Furthermore, acute pain activates the autonomic nervous system (ANS) and can induce a complex response characterized by hypertension, tachycardia, sweating, breathing alterations, restlessness, facial grimaces, alert behavior, pallor, and mydriasis.

Notably, if inadequately controlled, the pain symptom may persist beyond healing and become chronic pain. Generally, according to temporal criteria, a timeframe of 3 months is considered to define chronic pain. Generally, two types of pain are recognized: nociceptive and neuropathic. Somatic or visceral nociceptive pain arises from the activation of pain receptors in response to harmful stimuli and is typically related to tissue damage. Neuropathic pain, on the other hand, results from damage or dysfunction within the nervous system itself, leading to abnormal pain processing. Both nociceptive and neuropathic pain, if inadequately managed, can lead to significant alterations in the nervous system. These types of pain can trigger gene activation and induce functional and structural changes in the peripheral ganglia, the spinal cord, and supraspinal structures such as the brain and midbrain. These alterations are part of central

© The Author(s), under exclusive license to Springer Nature Switzerland AG 2024

M. Cascella, *Exploring AI in Pain Research and Management*,
https://doi.org/10.1007/978-3-031-78833-8_3

nervous system plasticity, which includes central sensitization. Neuroplasticity in this context is linked to changes in sensory processing and pain modulation, which can result in diminished pain inhibition, reduced activity of the antinociceptive system, and a decrease in the availability of endogenous analgesic mediators like endorphins. Significantly, there are forms of pain that are primarily chronic (primary chronic pain). In this scenario, nociplastic pain is a spectrum of chronic pain conditions, such as fibromyalgia or nonspecific back pain, in which impaired central pain modulation causes central sensitization and chronic pain in the absence of actual or threatened damage to tissues [2]. Therefore, beyond a temporal criterion, it is assumed that while acute pain may serve an adaptive role, chronic pain is maladaptive in nature as it "neither protects nor supports healing and repair" [3].

A key aspect of the IASP definition is the clear distinction between nociception and pain: "Pain cannot be inferred solely from activity in sensory neurons" [1]. Nociception refers to the physiological mechanism by which our body detects and responds to potentially harmful stimuli or noxious input. It is essentially the body's sensory system that involves the transmission of signals from nociceptors to the central nervous system, where the information is processed. The process of nociception is complex and involves the transduction of the stimulus into an electrical signal with the generation of an action potential, the conduction of the nervous impulse through first-order neurons (cell body in the dorsal ganglion) to reach the synapse with the second order neuron (medullary), transfer of information in the synapse between neurons of first and second order in the dorsal horn of the spinal cord by the release of excitatory neurotransmitters such as glutamate and/or modulatory neuropeptides (e.g., substance P and CGRP), the perception which is a conscious experience of pain, both in its sensorial aspect (location, character, and discrimination) and affective (emotional) and, finally, the modulation of the stimulus-response process both in the ascending course and, in response to the stimulus, according to descending inhibitory pathways [4]. On the other hand, the term "pain" refers to a subjective and multifaceted experience that arises from the interpretation and perception of these signals by the brain, encompassing not only the sensory aspect but also the emotional and cognitive dimensions. In other words, while nociception is a biological process, pain is a convolute psychophysical phenomenon that can vary greatly from person to person. The experience of pain can therefore be structured with biological, psychological, and social factors and although pain is an adaptive phenomenon, it may have adverse effects on function and social and psychological well-being [5].

Furthermore, the IASP underlines that the inability to express and communicate pain does not exclude its absence [1]. This aspect is of fundamental importance in individuals suffering from communication gaps, for example, due to neurocognitive problems [6]. Consequently, the complete evaluation of the pain symptom/disease is of fundamental importance in all care settings.

3.2 The Challenge of Pain Assessment

The clinical evaluation of the patient with pain follows two fundamental moments including the interview and the semiotic phase. The intensity of pain and its interference with daily life are assessed using rating scales. Unidimensional and multidimensional pain scales are usually used for pain assessment. Nevertheless, unidimensional evaluation, by implementing, for example, the 0–10 numeric rating scale (NRS) and the visual analog scale (VAS), has important limitations. While simple and immediate, this approach is susceptible to reporting bias due to psychosocial factors, including tendencies to catastrophize or underreport pain [7]. Multidimensional scales, on the other hand, are assessment tools used to evaluate and quantify various aspects of pain, considering that pain is a complex and subjective experience that encompasses more than just the intensity of physical discomfort. These scales such as the brief pain inventory (BPI) which assesses both the intensity and interference of pain in the last 24 h [8], and the McGill Pain Questionnaire [9], also available in a short-form instrument [10], consider multiple dimensions of pain, including sensory, emotional, cognitive, and social aspects. Although these tools are particularly useful in clinical settings to provide a comprehensive understanding of a patient's pain experience, they can fail to provide an objective and exhaustive measurement of pain [11]. The key limitations of multidimensional pain scales include their inherent limited specificity. This gap arises because some of these scales are intentionally crafted to provide a comprehensive overview of various facets of the pain experience. However, this broad approach may lack the necessary granularity to effectively assess and differentiate between specific types of pain or cater to the unique characteristics of distinct medical conditions.

Additionally, response bias is another noteworthy limitation. This bias can manifest when patients, out of concern or apprehension, consciously or unconsciously alter their responses to pain assessments. For instance, individuals may fear that reporting higher levels of pain could lead to an increase in prescribed medication or more aggressive treatment measures, influencing their self-reported pain scores [7]. To verify the reliability of the data the combined use of multidimensional questionnaires such as the BPI and the NRS scale can be proposed; additionally, tools such as the patient global impression of change (PGIC) to verify how the perception of pain has changed after treatment can be adopted, although even this strategy is affected by limitations [12].

3.3 The Pain Matrix, Its Questioning, and Functional Networks

The mechanistic study of pain phenomena must necessarily consider the anatomo-functional characteristics of the "classic" nociceptive pathways alongside all the centers that contribute to processing the signal at various levels in physiological conditions and following chronicization from multiple causes. Accumulating neuroimaging and neurophysiological evidence suggest that there are structural and functional neurophysiological brain abnormalities in individuals suffering from pain. These studies have demonstrated that it is not logically possible to identify a single brain area responsible for pain processing. Instead, pain involves a complex network of brain regions, defined as the "pain matrix." [13]. Therefore, the neural circuitry underlying pain involves the integration of information across multiple brain regions, which contributes to the diverse phenomenology of pain.

Given these premises, identifying the brain areas encompassing the matrix is a primary challenge. Studies have detected key brain areas that consistently respond to pain stimuli irrespective of the modality used to elicit nociceptive input, and are crucial for its sensory, cognitive, and emotional aspects. Among these, the thalamus acts as a relay station, transmitting pain signals from the periphery to the cerebral cortex. The anterior insular cortex, particularly the posterior insular cortex, is involved in processing thermal stimuli and is activated by both acute and chronic pain [14]. This activation highlights its role in the ongoing perception and modulation of pain over time. The primary and secondary somatosensory cortices (S1 and S2) are critical for the sensory-discriminative aspect of pain, allowing the brain to localize and interpret the intensity of painful stimuli. The anterior cingulate cortex (ACC) is associated with the affective-motivational dimension of pain, contributing to the emotional response and the motivational aspects of avoiding pain. Furthermore, the prefrontal cortex (PFC), especially the dorsolateral region, plays a significant role in the cognitive-evaluative aspect of pain. It is involved in the higher-order processing and regulation of pain, including decision-making, attention, and pain-related memory. In addition to these primary areas, other regions also contribute to the processing of pain. The periaqueductal gray (PAG) in the midbrain is crucial for the descending modulation of pain, helping to regulate pain sensitivity and providing analgesia. The nucleus accumbens, part of the brain's reward system, is involved in the emotional and motivational components of pain. The amygdala, known for its role in emotional processing, is also implicated in the affective dimensions of pain, influencing how pain is perceived and remembered. Additionally, the hippocampus and cerebellum are also involved in pain processing [15]. Together, these regions form a complex and dynamic network that underlies the multifaceted experience of pain, integrating sensory, emotional, and cognitive information to shape the overall perception and response to pain.

Nevertheless, this matrix encompasses various areas that participate not only in the perception of pain but also in other sensory, motor, and cognitive functions, often processing information simultaneously. In this view, researchers have conducted studies that challenge the traditional interpretation of the pain matrix [16]. For example, experiments have demonstrated that pain intensity can be entirely dissociated from the magnitude of responses in the pain matrix [17]. They have also shown that the magnitude of brain responses is strongly influenced by the context in which the stimulus appears, particularly its novelty. Moreover, using laser-evoked electroencephalogram (EEG) and functional magnetic resonance imaging (fMRI), it has been revealed that non-nociceptive stimuli, as well as stimuli not perceived as painful, can elicit cortical responses with a spatial distribution indistinguishable from that of the pain matrix [18]. Although pain and brain activity have frequently been correlated, a causal relationship between neuronal activity and pain sensation has yet to be established [16]. Significantly, in individuals with congenital insensitivity to pain, no differences have been observed in the magnitude of activation in pain matrix areas compared to controls [19].

In a classic structure–function paradigm, regardless of the pain matrix concept, it is crucial to understand how the human brain processes nociceptive sensory input and how this leads to the perception of pain. Additionally, it is essential to investigate how inflammation, injury, or sustained nociceptive input, which induce peripheral and central sensitization, result in neuroplastic changes that impact the clinical phenomenology of chronic pain [20].

Another aspect concerns the correlations between key networks and clinical manifestation as pain is thought to arise from imbalances between different functional networks. The self-representational default mode network (DMN) is a functional network that is active during rest. It is composed of the ventromedial PFC, posterior cingulate cortex (PCC), inferior parietal cortex (IPC), pregenual ACC, and precuneus and is involved in self-referential thoughts, daydreaming, and mind-wandering. DMN plays a role in introspection, mentation processes, memory retrieval, and planning for the future. In individuals with chronic pain, the DMN often shows disrupted connectivity [21]. This disruption may lead to an increased focus on pain and self-referential thoughts about pain, contributing to the persistence and exacerbation of pain symptoms. For example, it was demonstrated that DMN perturbation depends on years lived with back pain [22]. Nonetheless, DMN alterations have been also shown in acute pain [23]. Another network, the behavioral relevance encoding salience network (SN), helps in detecting and filtering salient stimuli, directing attention to important sensory inputs, and coordinating responses. It involves regions such as the anterior insula cortex and dorsal ACC. The SN becomes hyperactive in chronic pain conditions, leading to an increased sensitivity to pain signals. This hyperactivity can enhance the perception of pain and contribute to the development of central sensitization, where the nervous system becomes more responsive to pain stimuli [24]. The SN is functionally correlated to the goal-oriented frontoparietal central executive network (CEN) and both networks are anti-correlated to the DMN [25]. Therefore, according to the triple network model, used to investigate cognitive and affective disorders, it appears that pain is managed by three distinct yet interconnected networks, each encoding a different aspect of pain. The impact of the sensorial experience on these different networks collectively results in the multifaceted clinical picture of pain [26].

3.4 Automatic Pain Assessment

In this intricate context, the realm of pain assessment can be explored through different modalities, encompassing both behavioral and instrumental approaches, also leveraging the capabilities of artificial intelligence (AI) methodologies for comprehensive pain analysis. Consequently, investigations are directed toward the advancement of automatic pain assessment (APA) systems [27]. The aim is to isolate the nociceptive component of pain, by setting its weight within the perceived symptomatology.

The term APA refers to the set of research and clinical approaches primarily focused on providing an objective and quantifiable measure of pain, reducing in turn reliance on subjective self-reports. This aspect is of paramount importance to support patients who are unable to effectively communicate their pain levels, such as infants, non-verbal individuals, and patients with cognitive impairments. Moreover, APA can be implemented for continuous and real-time monitoring of pain levels, particularly in clinical settings where constant human observation is impractical; in this context, APA can enhance the ability to track and manage pain more effectively.

In addition to clinical benefits, APA can boost pain-related research by providing precise and consistent data, contributing to the development of better pain management therapies and interventions. Overall, the main purpose of APA is to support personalized medicine approaches by tailoring pain management strategies to individual needs based on objective assessments. The quantitative pain assessment (i.e., APA) can be combined with standard qualitative evaluations, through clinical assessments—even implementing telemedicine [28]—and questionnaires, for designing patient-centered (tailored) pain management processes.

Significantly, APA systems can harness the power of AI. These methodologies, including machine learning (ML) and deep learning (DL) strategies, play a crucial role in analyzing vast amounts of data derived from various sources, such as facial expressions, physiological signals, and vocal characteristics. The obtained models can be trained to recognize patterns and correlations that may not be apparent to human observers, thereby enabling the detection of subtle indicators of pain that might otherwise go unnoticed. Furthermore, AI-driven APA systems can continuously improve their accuracy and reliability through iterative learning processes. The embedding of feedback from clinical outcomes and patient reports can enable these systems to refine their models over time, enhancing their ability to assess pain with increasing precision. This adaptive capability is particularly valuable in dynamic clinical environments where patient conditions can change rapidly. This feature is of particular importance in pain medicine. For example, a typical pain phenomenon in cancer patients is breakthrough cancer pain, characterized by a sudden increase in pain despite a well-controlled background pain. AI-based APA methods could be developed to intercept or anticipate the occurrence of this distressing symptom. AI's role extends to integrating multimodal data, combining information from different sources to form a comprehensive picture of a patient's pain experience. In this scenario, unsupervised ML models could release clusters, by merging structured and unstructured data. Pain trajectories, the role of pharmacological and non-pharmacological therapies, and key issues such as opioid prescriptions [29] and misuse [30], could be exhaustively addressed.

This holistic approach not only has the potential to improve the accuracy of pain assessments but also seems to be suitable to reach the goal of personalized pain management strategies, ensuring that interventions are tailored to the unique needs of each patient. Since the National Institutes of Health (NIH) Biomarkers Definitions Working Group defines a "biomarker" as "a characteristic that is objectively measured and evaluated as an indicator of normal biological processes, pathogenic processes, or pharmacologic responses to a therapeutic intervention" [31], the ambitious goal of AI-based APA strategies is to depict the landscape of pain biomarkers.

3.5 Overview of Different APA Strategies

The term APA serves as an umbrella encompassing a broad range of research approaches and methods in pain assessment and analysis [27]. Therefore, the exploration of pain and its mechanisms involves a diverse array of strategies, each designed to target specific brain regions and their complex processing mechanisms. It is difficult to find a comprehensive classification.

A classification system based on the neurological and neurophysiological targets of these diverse modalities can provide a robust and meaningful categorization. In this context, the neocortex is involved in unraveling cognitive intricacies, the limbic brain delves into emotional nuances, and the reptilian brain—the oldest layer of the brain, formed by the brainstem, including the medulla, pons, cerebellum, midbrain, globus pallidus, and olfactory bulbs—reveals instinctual responses. Probably, this tripartite division better reflects the comprehensive nature of pain research, recognizing the interplay between cognition, emotion, and instinct. Furthermore, this multifaceted understanding not only enhances our theoretical knowledge but also paves the way for innovative therapeutic interventions that target specific facets of the intricate pain experience. These interventions can be tailored to address the cognitive, emotional, and instinctual (i.e., biosignal-based) components of pain (Fig. 3.1).

On the other hand, since pain processing engages multiple brain regions, it must be underscored that, while of practical application, this approach also has obvious limitations. For example, biosignals can be applied to the study of all three macro-areas. Moreover, imaging techniques such as functional magnetic resonance imaging (fMRI) can target different brain areas. Grouper et al. [32] demonstrated that high pain sensitivity can be correlated to the activation of neural circuits involved in the affective and motivational features of pain, but other pain-related brain connectomes (comprehensive maps of neural connections within the brain) involve the midbrain (e.g., the periaqueductal gray) [33] and cortical regions such as primary motor cortex (M1), supplementary motor area (SMA), primary (S1) and secondary (S2) somatosensory cortices [34]. Duerden et al. [35] conducted a meta-analysis on 2873 coordinate points and found that the cortices most frequently activated by noxious stimuli were the right anterior insula and anterior cingulate cortex. This was followed by the left insula, bilateral S2, prefrontal cortex, and the S1/posterior parietal cortex.

Consequently, these methodologies can be more easily divided into two main categories: (1) behavioral-based approaches, which include the study of facial

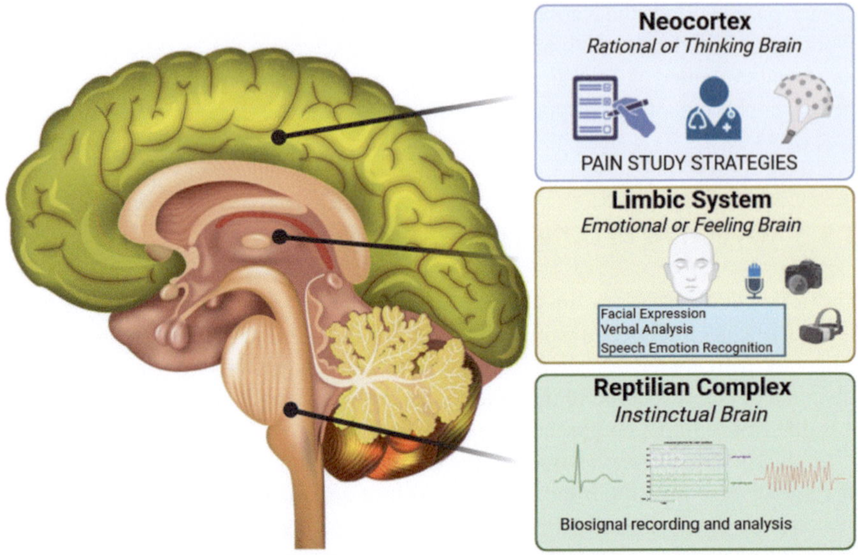

Fig. 3.1 Brain targets for APA research. Strategies for studying pain are categorized by the targeted brain regions and their processing mechanisms. The neocortex, particularly the somatosensory area, is crucial for understanding pain's location, intensity, and quality. Techniques such as imaging, EEG, and clinical examinations are used to investigate these mechanisms. The limbic system, the emotional center of the brain, is studied through behavioral approaches like facial expressions and speech emotion recognition. Lastly, the brainstem, the most ancient brain part, controls instinctual responses, with pain studies here focusing on recording and analyzing various biosignals

expressions, linguistic analyses, and non-verbal physical indicators of pain such as body movements; and (2) neurophysiology-based pain detection methods [27]. While this dichotomy is useful for narrative clarity, it is important to note that many approaches adopt multimodal strategies, integrating behavioral observations with neurophysiological techniques.

Furthermore, APA methods can be combined with other strategies that fall under objective pain assessment techniques. Many of these strategies focus on the precise characterization of pain or the underlying damage causing the pain. Electrophysiological studies can be included in this category; for example, quantitative sensory testing is a method used to evaluate sensory nerve function by applying controlled stimuli and measuring the sensory response. This approach helps quantify sensory pain thresholds for various types of stimuli, such as pressure, temperature, and vibration, providing valuable information about the nature and extent of sensory deficits or abnormalities associated with different pain conditions. Various types of stimuli are commonly used, including vibratory, thermal, and pressure stimuli. These stimuli activate peripheral receptors specific to each type of sensation, and the nerve fibers that innervate these receptors then transmit the sensation to the central nervous system [36].

3.5.1 Neurophysiology-Based Pain Detection Methods

This category includes biosignal investigations, functional imaging techniques, and other approaches, such as infrared thermometry.

3.5.1.1 Biosignals

Biosignals, which encompass a range of physiological data, are invaluable in understanding and managing pain. This set of physiological parameters, including heart rate variability (HRV) and other electrocardiogram (ECG)-derived biosignals, skin conductance parameters, as well as signals from brain activity such as electroencephalography (EEG), measure changes in response to pain by using minimally invasive or non-invasive technology. Some biosignals, such as EDA and HRV, reflect the activity of the autonomic nervous system, while others represent the overall functioning of organs or apparatus [27]. For example, EEG provides real-time insights into brain activity patterns and is utilized in both clinical and research contexts. However, this distinction is not without limitations. Take ECG as an example, cardiac activity is deeply influenced by the dynamic and fluctuating balance between the two arms of the autonomic system.

Most biosignals, such as ECG and EDA are collected by employing wearable sensors and devices.

3.5.1.1.1 Electroencephalography

EEG is a non-invasive method used to record the electrical activity of the brain. It involves placing electrodes on the scalp to detect the tiny electrical impulses produced by neurons. These impulses are then amplified and recorded, creating a visual representation of brain wave patterns.

The EEG signal is divided into four bands: alpha (8 – 13 Hz), which reflects a calm and balanced state of mind; beta (13 – 30 Hz), associated with emotional and cognitive processes, often linked to stress; delta (0.1 – 4 Hz), which is related to deep sleep stages and high activity in this range is seen as a sign of unconsciousness; and theta (4 – 8 Hz), which generates the theta rhythm, a neural oscillation connected to cognitive functions such as learning, memory, and spatial navigation.

Interestingly, EEG can serve as a promising tool for investigating "pain biomarkers" [37, 38]. Distinct neuronal activities in the sensorimotor cortex, such as elevations in theta and gamma oscillations, may correlate to specific pain states [39]. Furthermore, investigations conducted on resting-state EEG power in migraine, fibromyalgia, neuropathic pain, and spinal cord injury [40, 41] have shown increased theta power compared to healthy controls. This increase may be explained by the thalamocortical dysrhythmia theory, which suggests that heightened theta power is linked to impaired thalamic inhibition [42]. Other studies suggested that the gamma band predominantly predicts acute thermal pain and the peak alpha frequency recorded at the bilateral temporal scalp correlates with verbal pain reports during both stimulation and rest [43, 44].

Similarly to other biosignals, EEG is suitable for AI-based investigations. In a study, Chen et al. [45] introduced a multilayer CNN model for objective EEG-based pain detection. Ten volunteers participated in a series of 15 movement tasks (e.g., jogging on a running machine) and viewed 15 short videos depicting pain scenes. Following data acquisition and preprocessing, the model was validated on its ability to distinguish between "non-pain" and "pain" states, achieving an AUC ROC of 0.83 and 0.81 for the movement and video tasks, respectively.

Several other studies have explored EEG datasets using different ML approaches. Misra et al. [39] employed an SVM algorithm for binary classification (e.g., pain/no pain). Levitt et al. [37, 46] utilized SVM to obtain pain phenotypes from EEG features in individuals with chronic lumbar radiculopathy and those scheduled for neuromodulation therapy. Additionally, Nezam et al. [47] collected EEG and electromyogram (EMG) signals. They employed SVM and KNN decision tree models to evaluate different pain levels, achieving classification accuracies exceeding 80%. In another study, Elsayed et al. [48] combined signal processing techniques and ML strategies to analyze brain signals related to pain, categorizing them into four levels of pain intensity. Their classifier demonstrated an impressive accuracy of 94.83%. These findings, supported by other studies, suggest that normalized alpha power in the central brain region and other EEG signatures may serve as a reliable marker for chronic pain, with significant potential for clinical utility [49, 50]. Other investigations have been carried out. Vijayakumar et al. [50] used an RF approach to predict pain scores in healthy subjects, achieving high intrasubject and intersubject accuracies of 93% and 89.5%, respectively. Additionally, Vuckovic et al. [42, 51] used ANN, SVM, and linear discriminant analysis to identify spinal cord injured individuals at risk of developing central neuropathic pain, achieving accuracies surpassing 85% in all models. Finally, recent evidence suggests that EEG features can predict the effects of pain treatments, further highlighting the potential of EEG in pain assessment and management [52].

3.5.1.1.2 Electrocardiography-Derived Biosignals

The ECG signal records the superficial electrical activity of the heart. Temporal variations in inter-beat intervals offer a measure of HRV, which is closely tied to the functioning of the autonomic nervous system (ANS) [53]. HRV is influenced by the dynamic interplay between the sympathetic and parasympathetic branches of the ANS, known as sympathovagal balance. These branches work antagonistically to regulate heart rate according to the body's changing requirements. Alterations in this equilibrium, reflected in HRV fluctuations, can result from physiological factors (e.g., circadian rhythm) and pathological conditions (such as diabetes and post-infarction situations) [54]. These fluctuations can also indicate physiological responses to stress and pain scenarios [20]. The RR series, representing the intervals between successive R waves of the QRS complex on the ECG waveform, can be computed to extract time-domain HRV parameters. HRV reflects the balance between the sympathetic and parasympathetic nervous systems. Increased sympathetic activity leads to a "fight or flight" response, which prepares the body for rapid action. This results in decreased HRV where the intervals between heartbeats become more uniform (less variability), as the heart rate generally increases to prepare the body for action. On the contrary, increased parasympathetic activity is associated with "rest and digest" functions, promoting relaxation and recovery. This results in increased HRV featuring more variability in the time intervals between heartbeats. A higher HRV indicates a healthy and responsive cardiovascular system, capable of adapting to a wide range of conditions. Several HRV metrics can be used, such as the standard deviation of RR intervals (SDRR) and the root mean square of successive differences (RMSSD).

More sophisticated ECG-derived features, including spectral analysis and non-linear measures, can provide deeper insights into the heart's response to pain. Techniques such as the analysis of power spectral density and fractal dimensions of HRV, for example, can reveal subtle changes in autonomic regulation associated with different pain states. In this scenario, the analgesia nociception index (ANI), which ranges from 0 to 100, is a commercialized tool derived from HRV for pain evaluation during surgery [55].

3.5.1.1.3 Electrodermal Activity

EDA measures changes in the electrical properties of the skin, typically associated with sweat gland activity. While it is mostly measured on the palmar surface, EDA can also be recorded at other sites, such as the soles of the feet, fingers, or forehead. Activation of the sympathetic nervous system, such as during stress, excitement, or anxiety, prompts an increase in sweat production, even without physical exertion. This signal is an indicator of sympathetic nervous system activity and is considered an indicator of emotions and arousal [56]. Therefore, it has been efficiently applied in tasks related to pain recognition [57] and other aims. Combined with other bio-signals, it has been also integrated into investigations that implement games and virtual reality technology [58].

This approach serves as a valuable marker for assessing pain-induced neurocognitive stress by detecting alterations in the electrical properties of the skin, stemming from sweat gland activation, and resulting in an elevation in skin conductance. The continuous variations in skin conductance are termed the skin conductance level (SCL); it is the tonic component with a more gradual change, representing the overall level of arousal. On the other hand, the phasic component captures the brief changes in the EDA signal; it is the skin conductance response (SCR) triggered by the presentation of a stimulus. SCR is a rapid, temporary increase in skin conductance in response to stimuli. The frequency of SCR varies between 0.05 and 1–2 Hz. Both SCL and SCT contribute to defining the whole skin conductance. Typically, the EDA signal is quantified in microsiemens (μS): the amplitude of SCR peaks commonly ranges between 0.1 and 1 μS, whereas the amplitude of SCL ranges between 2 and 20 μS (Fig. 3.2).

3.5.1.1.4 Electromyography and Surface Electromyography

Electromyography (EMG) is a technique used to measure and record the electrical activity of muscles. It involves inserting small needles or electrodes into the muscle tissue to detect electrical signals generated by muscle contractions. For APA research, EMG can be used to investigate behavior (movements) in individuals suffering from chronic pain (e.g., low back pain) [59]. Surface EMG (sEMG) is a

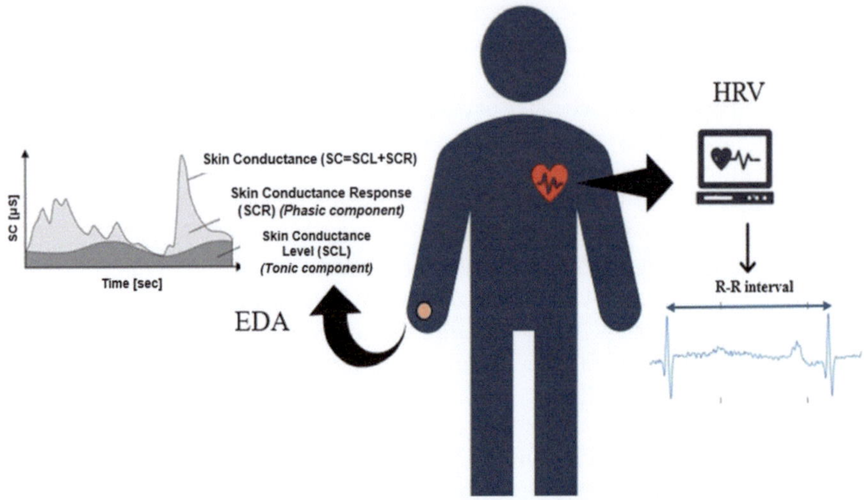

Fig. 3.2 Electrodermal activity (EDA) and heart rate variability (HRV). Changes in skin conductance (SC) over time are featured by a tonic component (skin conductance level, SCL) and a phasic component (skin conductance response, SCR) (left side). EDA measures changes in the electrical properties of the skin, often linked to sweat gland activity (here the palmar surface). When the sympathetic nervous system is activated (e.g., during stress, excitement, or anxiety), it triggers an increase in sweat production, even in the absence of physical exertion. This leads to higher skin conductance levels. HRV is a measure of the variation in time between consecutive heartbeats, known as R-R intervals (right side). It decreases with sympathetic activation (indicating stress or exertion) and increases with parasympathetic activation (indicating relaxation and recovery)

non-invasive variant of EMG. Instead of using needle electrodes, surface electrodes are placed on the skin over the superficial muscle. It is implemented for tasks like monitoring muscle function during movement or rehabilitation exercises [60]. Furthermore, sEMG is an emerging technology in automatic pattern recognition. This technique seems to be particularly advantageous for detecting subtle facial muscle activity that might not be visible to the naked eye. However, an evidence-based review identified only one study that used sEMG to objectively detect facial pain expressions [61]. Consequently, the proposed correlation between muscle tension and pain intensity necessitates further investigation [62].

3.5.1.1.5 Photoplethysmography

Photoplethysmography (PPG) is a non-invasive optical technique used to measure variations in blood volume through the use of a light source and a corresponding photodetector. The process involves illuminating a portion of the body's surface, such as the skin and underlying blood vessels, with light. The photodetector then captures the variations in the light that are either reflected or transmitted, depending on the design of the PPG sensor. These variations are influenced by the pulsatile nature of blood flow, which is affected by factors including heartbeats, blood vessel elasticity, and respiratory rate. Recent advancements in PPG technology have led to the development of automatic classifiers designed to detect PPG pulses with greater accuracy. These classifiers analyze the unique morphological features of the PPG signals, which reflect the pulse waveform and its distinctive characteristics [63]. PPG can be employed for more sophisticated analyses. For example, Cao et al. [64] utilized photoplethysmography (PPG) to extract potential pain-related respiratory features from postoperative patients participating in the UCI iHurtDB pain protocol [65]. They applied five machine learning algorithms—ADABoost, XGBoost, random forest, SVM, and KNN classifiers—and achieved satisfactory accuracy with each. The authors compared their findings with those of Thiam and Schwenker [66], who used 65 automatic respiratory features and employed an appropriate fusion architecture method.

3.5.1.1.6 Pupillometry

Pupil dilation, a response of the sympathetic nervous system to acute pain, has been demonstrated to correlate with the intensity of controlled noxious stimuli [67]. While pupil diameter at rest is predominantly influenced by ambient light and shows no correlation with pain levels, dynamic pupillary measures can provide insights into ongoing pain in conscious subjects. These measures include the pupillary light reflex and spontaneous pupil diameter fluctuations. These fluctuations can be quantified using two distinct measures: pupillary unrest under ambient light (PUAL) and the variation coefficient of pupillary diameter. PUAL involves monitoring the natural, minute oscillations in pupil size that occur under constant ambient lighting conditions. These fluctuations reflect the underlying autonomic nervous system activity and can provide an indirect measure of pain intensity. The PUAL technique involves using an eye tracking device to record continuous pupil size measurements while the subject is in a stable light environment. The recorded data is then analyzed to identify patterns and quantify the amplitude and frequency of pupil size changes. Therefore, this strategy can help capture subtle changes in autonomic nervous system activity that may be missed by static measurements of pupil diameters. Despite promising results, researchers failed to prove the efficacy of pupillometry in evaluating acute pain.

3.5.1.1.7 Accelerometry

Accelerometer signals capture motor activity along the three primary axes of an orthogonal Cartesian plane, providing detailed measurements of movement in three dimensions. These signals have been shown to correlate with stress-induced pain in patients, making them a valuable tool for assessing the physical manifestations of pain. An accelerometer usually contains a microelectromechanical system (MEMS), which consists of a small mass suspended inside the device. When the device moves, the mass shifts and this movement is converted into an electrical signal that corresponds to acceleration. Accelerometry can be used to quantify motion-associated pain and physical activity in individuals suffering from chronic pain [68].

Inertial measurement unit (IMU) is a more advanced type of motion-sensing device that combines multiple sensors to provide comprehensive data on an object's orientation, velocity, and acceleration. An IMU typically includes an accelerometer, providing data on how fast an object is moving in any direction, a gyroscope that measures angular velocity or the rate of rotation around the X-, Y-, and Z-axes and, occasionally, a magnetometer. The latter measures the strength and direction of magnetic fields, often used to provide heading information relative to the Earth's magnetic north. IMUs are essential in autonomous vehicles for navigation, in drones for stable flight, in smartphones for enhanced motion detection, and in virtual reality systems for tracking user movements. This technology was also applied to categorize nonspecific low back pain patients by means an ML approach [69].

3.5.1.1.8 Biosignal Acquisition and Processing

For acquiring and analyzing biosignals, it is essential to use validated strategies that encompass the processes of signal acquisition, signal processing, and signal analysis. This aspect is crucial within the research framework. Physiological signals like EMG, ECG, and SCL are highly susceptible to various types of noise (such as thermal and powerline interference) and artifacts. Therefore, these data typically undergo a preprocessing phase to minimize or eliminate the impact of unwanted noise and other environmental factors.

In the case of EDA biosignals, different types of analysis can be performed such as continuous decomposition analysis (CDA) and trough-to-peak (TTP) analysis. CDA separates SCR and SCL by deconvolving the skin conductance data with its impulse response function over time. This process allows for the estimation of both tonic and phasic activity from the deconvolution results.

Regarding the analysis of accelerometer data, the magnitude of acceleration can be derived from the raw XYZ acceleration signals and utilized as a comprehensive metric to capture significant changes in overall acceleration, independent of the device's orientation. The accelerometer records the acceleration forces as the subject moves. These forces are recorded along three axes—X (left-right), Y (forward-backward), and Z (up-down)—capturing the intensity and direction of the movements. The raw data collected by the accelerometer consists of continuous signals representing the acceleration in each direction. These data can include noise or constant effects like gravity, which need to be filtered out. The resulting acceleration signal can be then filtered for example by using a Butterworth bandpass filter (or maximally flat magnitude filter), for example with cut-off frequencies of 0.25 Hz and 2.5 Hz [68]. The filtered accelerometry data is then analyzed to extract meaningful information, such as the magnitude of movements, frequency, and patterns. In particular, the acceleration vector magnitude (Acc) can be calculated using the following eq. [70]:

$$\text{Acc magnitude} = \sqrt{a^2_{\ x} + a^2_{\ y} + a^2_{\ z}}$$

where ax, ay, and az represent the acceleration on the x-, y-, and z-axes, respectively. The final acceleration vector magnitude can be refined by subtracting the mean to eliminate constant effects like gravity [70] (Fig. 3.3).

Even EMG signals can be filtered (e.g., in the range 20 Hz to 250 Hz) using a Butterworth bandpass filter. For ECG-derived analyses, R peaks are usually detected

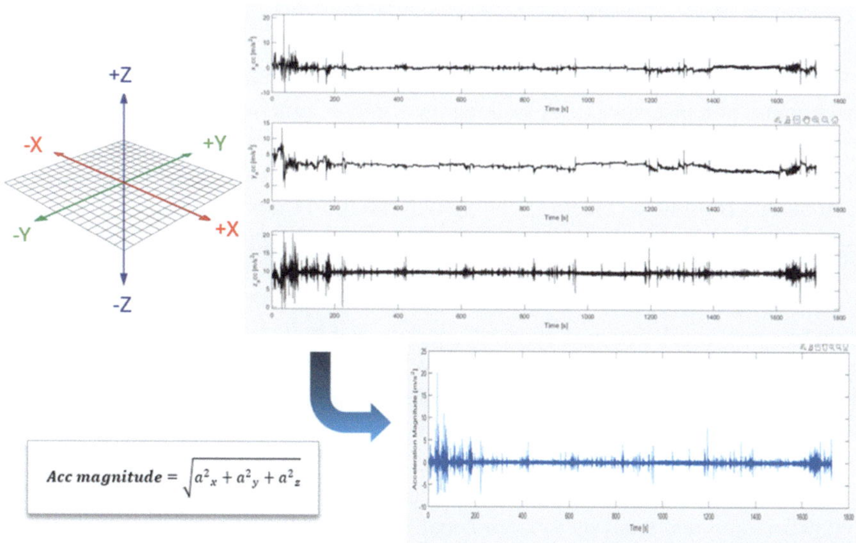

Fig. 3.3 The accelerometer captures movement by recording acceleration forces along three axes: X (left-right), Y (forward-backward), and Z (up-down). This raw data consists of continuous signals indicating the acceleration in each direction. By filtering and analyzing this data, meaningful insights can be extracted. The overall acceleration, or acceleration vector magnitude (Acc), is calculated using the formula in the box, where ax, ay, and az represent the accelerations on the X-, Y-, and Z-axes, respectively. From the author

using a modified Pan-Tompkins technique [71]. This approach involves analyzing the ECG envelope and flattening the signal to enhance the QRS complexes. The raw series of intervals between consecutive R peaks (R-R intervals) is then extracted. Next, a recursive filtering process is applied to the R-R time series to eliminate outliers and intervals that deviate significantly from the mean of adjacent R-R intervals. High- and low-frequency noises are then removed by filtering. From this filtered R-R time series, the heart rate (HR) time series is derived. The standard deviation (SD) of both the R-R intervals and the HR series is then calculated and used as a time-domain measure of HRV [72].

Table 3.1 provides the examples of various types of EDA and ECG biosignals, and the parameters used.

Additionally, many techniques can be utilized to extract features and build classification models from physiological signals for deep learning applications. For instance, researchers proposed a multimodal Deep Denoising Convolutional AutoEncoders (DDCAE) architecture that employs CNNs. This method effectively reduced the sampling rate, noise, and artifacts from EDA, ECG, and EMG signals while incorporating data augmentation. In the DDCAE model, a gating layer generates a weighted representation based on the latent features from each input channel, optimizing an inference model for classification or regression tasks. An attention mechanism was also applied; it focuses on the most relevant parts of the input data to create a more accurate weighted representation and thereby enhances overall performance [73].

Several wearable non-invasive devices are available for acquiring EDA and other biosignals. For instance, EDA is integrated into Internet-of-Things (IoT) devices such as the BITalino® multi-channel platform. This open-source biosignal platform is compatible with user-friendly software like OpenSignals, enabling the acquisition of data from ECG, electromyography (EMG), EDA, and EEG.

Another device is the Empatica E4 Wristband (Empatica Inc., Boston, MA, USA), designed for recording EDA and PPG. This wristband also measures heart rate, motion-based activity (via accelerometer data on the x-, y-, and z-axes), and skin temperature. It features an event-marking tag button and is primarily used in research fields such as psychology, neuroscience, and physiology. Additionally, the Empatica E4 is employed for monitoring stress and emotional states, tracking sleep patterns, and physical activity in chronic pain rehabilitation [74].

Concerning software, most EDA data analysis is performed with custom-written scripts in MATLAB. However, some studies have focused on developing EDA signal processing and analysis tools to benefit researchers without specialized expertise. For example, Bach et al. [75] introduced a MATLAB software called SCRalyze, which is based on general convolution modeling. Additionally, Benedek and Kaernbach developed Ledalab, a MATLAB-compatible software that employs discrete and CDA [76]. Furthermore, Greco et al. [77] developed cvxEDA, a software that uses the cvxEDA method and is compatible with both Python and MATLAB. For

Table 3.1 Example of features calculated through the analysis of EDA and ECG signals

Type of Signal	Features
Electrodermal activity (EDA)	**Features from continuous decomposition analysis (CDA)** • Number of significant skin conductance responses (nTTP) [a.u.] • Maximum value of skin conductance responses (maxCDA) [μS] • Minimum value of skin conductance responses (minCDA) [μS] • Mean value of skin conductance responses (meanCDA) [μS] • Maximum interval between skin conductance responses (maxDiffTTP) [ms] • Minimum interval between skin conductance responses (minDiffTTP) [ms] • Mean interval between skin conductance responses (meanDiffTTP) [ms] **Features from trough-to-peak analysis (TTP)** • Number of significant skin conductance responses (nTTP) [a.u.] • Maximum value of skin conductance responses (maxTTP) [μS] • Minimum value of skin conductance responses (minTTP) [μS] • Mean value of skin conductance responses (meanTTP) [μS] • Maximum interval between skin conductance responses (maxDiffTTP) [ms] • Minimum interval between skin conductance responses (minDiffTTP) [ms] • Mean interval between skin conductance responses (meanDiffTTP) [ms]

Table 3.1 (continued)

Type of Signal	Features
Electrocardiography (ECG)	**Features from time-domain analysis (TDA) of heart rate variability (HRV)** • Mean value of RR intervals (mRR) [ms] • Standard deviation of RR intervals (SDRR) [ms] • Mean value of heart rate (mHR) [bpm] • Standard deviation of HR (SDHR) [bpm] • Root mean square of successive differences of RR intervals (RMSSD) [ms] Number of successive RR intervals <50 ms (NN50) [a.u.] Percentage of successive RR intervals <50 ms (pNN50) [%] **Features from frequency domain analysis (FDA) of heart rate variability (HRV)** • Peak value in the very low-frequency band of the HRV power density spectrum (peakVLF) [Hz] • Peak value in the low-frequency band of the HRV power density spectrum (peakLF) [Hz] • Peak value in the high-frequency band of the HRV power density spectrum (peakHF) [Hz] • Power in the very low-frequency band of the HRV power density spectrum (powVLF) [ms^2] • Power in the low-frequency band of the HRV power density spectrum (powLF) [ms^2] • Power in the high-frequency band of the HRV power density spectrum (powHF) [ms^2] • Total power of the HRV power density spectrum (Ptot) [ms^2] • Percentage power in the very low-frequency band of the HRV power density spectrum concerning the total power (%VLF) [%] • Percentage power in the low-frequency band of the HRV power density spectrum for the total power (%LF) [%] • Percentage power in the high-frequency band of the HRV power density spectrum for the total power (%HF) [%] • Normalized power in the low-frequency band of the HRV power density spectrum for the sum of LF and HF power (nLF) [a.u.] • Normalized power in the high-frequency band of the HRV power density spectrum for the sum of LF and HF power (nHF) [a.u.] • Sympathovagal balance measured as the ratio between power in LF and power in the LF band (LF/HF) [a.u]

EDA noise and artifact detection, Taylor et al. [78] created an open-source program named EDA Explorer, which uses SVMs for data analysis and is compatible only with Python.

3.5.1.2 Functional Imaging Techniques

Functional Magnetic Resonance Imaging (fMRI) is a powerful neuroimaging set of techniques used to observe and measure brain activity by detecting changes in blood flow. Usually, fMRI employs the Blood Oxygen Level Dependent (BOLD) signal, which reflects changes in blood oxygenation levels. Oxygen levels in the blood influence the MRI signal because oxygenated and deoxygenated blood have distinct magnetic properties that can be detected by MRI [78]. The BOLD technique in fMRI is highly effective for studying acute and experimental pain, where there are brief periods of pain followed by periods without pain, leading to rapidly changing hemodynamic responses. This capability was employed to examine acute pain responses in pain-free volunteers as well as in patients with chronic pain. However, BOLD fMRI is less suited for monitoring responses to persistent or chronic pain conditions due to its limited ability to capture sustained changes over time. For chronic pain or persistent pain conditions, an alternative fMRI technique, known as arterial spin labeling (ASL), is more appropriate. ASL provides a direct measure of cerebral blood flow by using magnetically labeled endogenous water in the blood as a diffusible tracer. Unlike BOLD, which is sensitive to rapid changes in blood oxygenation, ASL offers improved quantification of regional blood flow, resulting in a more accurate estimation of ongoing cerebral perfusion. A specific advanced form of ASL is 3D Pulsed Arterial Spin Labeling (PASL) MRI, which is used to map cerebral perfusion. Different studies have been conducted to evaluate the technique in pain conditions, such as chronic knee pain [79], fibromyalgia [80], neuropathic pain [81], and post-surgical pain [82]. Another technique, pseudo-continuous ASL (pCASL), utilizes a continuous sequence of radiofrequency pulses to magnetically label arterial blood water. This method provides more continuous and precise labeling of blood flow compared to earlier ASL techniques. Another approach includes the ultra-high-field (UHF) 7 T-MRI, which features an augmented signal-to-noise ratio and increased sensitivity in BOLD contrast change. These properties can limit nonspecific mapping signals from large vessels and accentuate microvasculature contributions [83].

Researchers have attempted to simultaneously record EEG and fMRI responses to noxious stimuli. This approach aims to combine the high temporal resolution of EEG with the high spatial resolution of fMRI. Nevertheless, interpreting these studies requires caution, as EEG and fMRI may not sample the same neural activity. Simultaneous EEG-fMRI is the term for using both methods concurrently [84]. This approach is valuable for evaluating the correlation between the brain's electrical activity and the hemodynamic changes that occur on macro and micro scales. While fMRI provides high spatial resolution, it lacks precise temporal resolution due to the slow BOLD signal, which responds in seconds. Conversely, EEG offers high temporal resolution with millisecond response latency but has poor spatial localization. By integrating fMRI and EEG, a synergy is achieved, enhancing the detail and accuracy of observing the brain's responses to noxious stimuli. Warbrick [85] dissected the current state and prospects of combining EEG and fMRI methods. The author addressed several key aspects, including the importance of average artifact subtraction (AAS) for obtaining a clean EEG signal and dealing with pulse-related artifacts. Briefly, two main approaches can be adopted to integrate EEG-fMRI data: symmetric and asymmetric. In asymmetric approaches, information from one modality is used to predict the other, whereas symmetric approaches can be either model-driven or data-driven.

3.5.1.3 Functional Near-Infrared Spectroscopy

Functional near-infrared spectroscopy (fNIRS) is a non-invasive imaging technique that detects concentration changes in oxygenated hemoglobin (HbO) and deoxygenated hemoglobin (HbR), similar to the BOLD signal in fMRI. fNIRS operates by measuring the absorption of near-infrared light at wavelengths between 700 and 1000 nm, which penetrates the skull and underlying brain tissue [86]. The process involves emitting near-infrared light through the scalp and detecting the light that is either absorbed or scattered by the brain tissue. Changes in the concentration of HbO and HbR alter the absorption properties of the tissue, allowing the device to infer brain activity based on hemodynamic responses associated with neural activation [87].

Unlike MRI scanners, fNIRS systems are portable and can be easily transported to different locations, making them suitable for a variety of research and clinical environments. Furthermore, fNIRS does not require a large, static magnetic field, allowing it to be used in settings where MRI's strong magnetic field would interfere with other equipment. For example, this property makes fNIRS particularly useful in surgical environments where various electrical and ferromagnetic tools are in use. Moreover, fNIRS equipment is generally less expensive than MRI machines, making it a more accessible option for many research and clinical institutions.

In neuroscience research, fNIRS is widely used to study brain function in various cognitive tasks, such as language processing, motor activities, and social interactions. Researchers can monitor brain activity in naturalistic settings outside the constraints of an MRI scanner. For clinical diagnostics, the technique is implemented for diagnosing and monitoring neurological conditions such as stroke, traumatic brain injury, and neurodevelopmental disorders. It is also used for intraoperative monitoring as well as in combination with EEG featuring hybrid frameworks [88].

There are different limitations. While fNIRS provides good temporal resolution, its spatial resolution is lower compared to fMRI. Additionally, the near-infrared light used in fNIRS can only penetrate a few centimeters into the brain, limiting its ability to measure deep brain structures. However, it is effective for cortical surface imaging. Yet, the signals obtained from fNIRS are influenced by various factors, including skin and skull thickness, and extracerebral blood flow. More recent approaches such as time-domain fNIRS (TD fNIRS) and continuous wave fNIRS offer improved sensitivity to the brain hemodynamics [89].

Given its properties, the technique has been also utilized for pain research. For example, in a study involving patients with hypersensitive teeth, researchers employed fNIRS to measure hemodynamic cortical responses while the patients were seated in a dental chair. They identified distinct hemodynamic activity in the S1 and PFCs triggered by thermal stimulation of the affected tooth, from the anticipation of pain to its perception. Notably, the patients' clinical pain experiences were predicted by their baseline functional connectivity between the S1 and PFC, along with a clear sequence of hemodynamic responses. This process, involving both sensory-discriminative and cognitive-emotional components, started during the anticipation of pain (pre-pain phase) with activations in the contralateral S1 orofacial region and bilateral PFC. Interestingly, these activations were then followed by either flat or deactivation in the PFC and further responses in the S1 when the cold stimuli became painful (pain phase) [90, 91]. Other recent examples of application in pain research regard the study of the primary motor area activity in the phantom limb phenomenon [92], the evaluation of therapeutic methods for addressing chronic low back pain [93], and pain assessment during acupuncture [94].

3.5.1.4 Infrared Thermography and Other Strategies

Infrared thermography (IRT) can be implemented for APA. Given that the skin is the body's largest organ, it plays a crucial role in the diagnostic process. IRT imaging captures temperature variations on the skin's surface, producing infrared thermograms that reflect the underlying physiology of peripheral blood flow, which is regulated by the autonomic nervous system. Consequently, temperature recordings can quantify shifts in sympathetic tension, often resulting from injury or other pathological conditions. In particular, this method measures thermal energy exchange between a body and its surroundings by capturing infrared radiation within the wavelength range of 0.78 μm to 1 mm in the electromagnetic spectrum. By analyzing these infrared emissions, IRT provides detailed thermal images that reflect variations in temperature across the surface of an object or body. This capability allows for precise monitoring of thermal patterns, which can be used to assess physiological processes, detect abnormalities, and evaluate various conditions based on thermal changes.

Two types of thermographic techniques are available: passive thermography and active thermography. Passive thermography uses a thermal camera without any external thermal excitation system, simply measuring the temperature of the object. In contrast, active thermography involves external excitation systems to stimulate the skin and body, allowing for the measurement of their thermal response over time. The active approach has been used, for instance, for cancer diagnosis [95]. In healthy individuals, there is typically a high degree of thermal symmetry between the two sides of the body, with a normal temperature difference of about 0.5 ± 0.3 °C [96]. Deviations from this symmetry, such as asymmetric thermal patterns, may indicate the presence of disease such as in stroke [97]. Previous research has also established a connection between pain and autonomic dysfunction, which can manifest as alterations in skin temperature. The use of IRT for diagnosing lumbosacral radicular pain is based on the principle that compression or irritation of nerve roots can influence sympathetic nerve activity. This, in turn, affects vasomotor control and leads to changes in skin temperature [98]. Attention must be given to minimizing interference from external infrared sources, lighting, and background conditions. For instance, external lighting and radiating sources can cause temperature readings to deviate by approximately 1.5 °C. It is also advisable to avoid using air conditioning units during the measurement process. Additionally, it is recommended that the patient remain at rest for 20–30 min before measurements to allow their body to acclimate to the ambient environmental conditions. While several case studies have been conducted to demonstrate the diagnostic potential of thermography in assessing pain, several open issues remain. They concern the clinical setting to be investigated as well as the exact definition of research pathways and protocols.

Other APA strategies are available, although less investigated. For instance, Schmidt et al. [99] used nociceptive electrical stimulation on the hands of healthy individuals to study eye movements during different tasks of visual exploration. Their research on eye tracking demonstrated that pain influences attentional shifts, leading to fewer saccades and longer fixations, indicative of reduced exploratory behavior. However, as noted by the authors, the implications of these findings for chronic pain conditions remain unclear.

3.5.2 Behavioral-Based Approaches for APA

In recent years, the integration of behavioral-based approaches has significantly advanced the field of APA. These methods leverage observable behavioral cues, such as facial expressions, speech analysis, and other methods. Notably, various AI approaches have been proposed to enhance the accuracy and reliability of these assessments.

3.5.2.1 Facial Expressions

Facial expressions play a pivotal role in non-verbal communication, particularly in conveying pain to others. Moreover, facial expressions of pain demonstrate consistency across various factors, including age, gender, cognitive states (e.g., noncommunicative patients), and different types of pain [100]. They may even correlate with self-reported pain levels. As a result, extensive research has been dedicated to studying facial expressions as indicators of pain behavior, enabling automatic and objective pain assessment and the existence of facial activity patterns that are associated with pain has been postulated [101, 102].

Facial expressions indicative of pain can be categorized into two types: voluntary and involuntary physical manifestations. While voluntary expressions are consciously initiated by the cortex and can be controlled in real-time, they tend to be less fluid and display more variability in movement. Involuntary facial expressions, on the other hand, are unconsciously triggered by subcortical processes and are characterized by symmetrical, synchronized, reflex-like movements of facial muscles, giving them a seamless appearance.

Action Units (AUs) are referral elements for studying this behavior. They are specific facial muscle movements or activations used to describe and analyze facial expressions. The concept of AUs was introduced in 1978 by psychologists Paul Ekman and Wallace V. Friesen as part of their Facial Action Coding System (FACS), which serves as a comprehensive tool for describing and analyzing human facial expressions [103]. FACS defines and categorizes 46 individual AUs, each representing a distinct movement or combination of movements of facial muscles, such as raising the eyebrows, wrinkling the nose, or pursing the lips. The Prkachin and Solomon Pain Intensity (PSPI) is a pain expression score based on FACS. The authors conducted a benchmark study on pain-related action units (AUs) using images from 129 individuals experiencing shoulder pain. They assessed facial expressions of pain during induced acute pain through motion analysis. Following Ekman's coding system, four certified human coders evaluated each image, classifying pain intensity on a scale from 1 (trace) to 5 (maximum). The study identified six AUs significantly associated with pain: brow lowering (AU4), orbital tightening (AU6 and AU7), levator contraction (AU9 and AU10), and eye closure (AU43) [104].

Manual analysis of this process can be highly intricate, but with the emergence of AI techniques, there has been a shift toward computer-mediated automatic detection of pain-related behaviors, employing various AI-based image processing strategies. AI-driven systems can analyze facial expressions in real time, providing consistent and objective evaluations that reduce the subjectivity inherent in human assessment. These systems utilize ML algorithms to identify and classify AUs (or other features) associated with pain, enabling healthcare providers to monitor pain levels accurately and respond appropriately.

Diverse strategies have been implemented in terms of feature selection, signal processing, and algorithms implemented [102]. Different automated facial recognition algorithms such as Facereader7©, OpenFace©, and Affdex SDK© as well as AI architectures can be used. In a recent investigation focused on cancer pain, we conducted a brief interview lasting approximately 2 min alongside a video recording. The Delaware Pain Database and the UNBC-McMaster Shoulder Pain dataset [105] were used for training. A set of 17 AUs was adopted. The OpenFace toolkit was used to extract these AUs from each image. For continuous estimation, the entire patient video, with frame prediction values of 0 (no pain) or 1 (pain), was imported into an annotator (ELAN 6.4). The developed neural network classifier consisted of two dense layers. The first layer contained 17 nodes corresponding to the facial AUs extracted by OpenFace© for each image. The output layer provided a classification label of "pain" (1) or "no pain" (0). The classifier achieved an accuracy of approximately 94% after about 400 training epochs, with a ROC AUC value of approximately 0.98 [106].

Obviously, for this task, different challenges must be addressed. They mostly include the accurate selection of AUs, the architecture implemented, the data used for training and testing, and features processing. Concerning the latter issue, for example, Gomutbutra et al. [107] applied an innovative approach. They used OpenFace© to generate time series data for each action unit, capturing the facial movements of patients over time. This data was then transformed into two key metrics including the average movement intensity and the area AUC surrounding the maximum peak. To calculate the AUC for each action unit, they analyzed data from 22 frames (0.03 s per frame) around the maximum peak. Figure 3.4 shows frames from a CNN-based model.

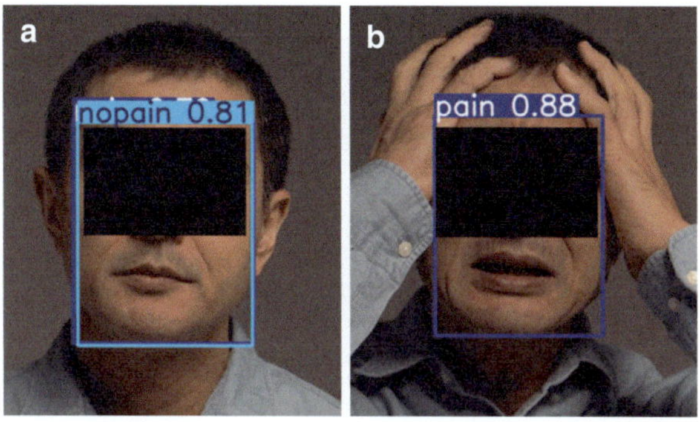

Fig. 3.4 The CNN was trained to recognize patterns and features from a set of AUs, enabling it to predict the patient's pain status based on their facial expressions in real-time. In the selected frames, the model recognized the absence of pain (**a**) and pain occurrence (**b**) with accuracy of 0.81 and 0.88, respectively. From the author

While AUs are the primary focus of many studies, alternative research pathways can also be employed to investigate this behavior. Zhi et al. [108] introduced a multimodal model that combines dynamic facial expression analysis with dynamic biomedical signal analysis. In their approach, facial expression analysis was based on distance features and head pose estimation. They calculated ten different distances between various facial features to identify pain-related actions such as lowering the brows, tightening the eyelids, closing the eyes, raising the cheeks and upper lip, wrinkling the nose, and stretching and opening the mouth. For head pose estimation, they measured three Euler angles—pitch, roll, and yaw—to track pain-related head movements like looking up and down, tilting sideways, and rotating left and right. The core concept involved rotating a 3D standard model to align the "2D projection" of its "3D landmarks" with the 2D landmarks in test images as closely as possible, with the rotation angle representing the head pose estimation. For this complex modeling, accurate preprocessing is of paramount importance. A typical approach to image preprocessing provides that images are initially aligned using rotation and scale transformations based on eye positions. The images are then cropped to a specified pixel size, and finally, an elliptical face region was isolated for feature extraction [109]. A different approach consists of cropping the face, extracting the face mask with landmarks, and frontalizing the mask using piecewise affine warping to align it with a standard image. The dataset can be also enhanced through landmark-based random deformations [110]. Feature extraction methods for assessing pain through facial expressions can be categorized into frame-level and sequence-level techniques. Frame-level feature extraction methods, which are widely used, include texture-based methods such as local binary patterns and wavelet-based methods like Gabor filters. Frame-level recognition is advantageous due to its simplicity, low complexity, and ease of application [111]. However, it is limited by the information available in a single image, missing dynamic details such as blinking. Sequence-level methods, on the other hand, capture the entire process of facial pain expression, providing more dynamic information, which is more relevant for clinical applications [112].

Advancements in AI and computer vision have led to the development of sophisticated tools capable of recognizing subtle changes in facial expressions that may indicate pain. These tools can be integrated into clinical settings to assist in the continuous monitoring of patients, particularly those who are unable to communicate their pain verbally [113].

3.5.2.2 Speech Analysis

Speech analysis involves studying and examining spoken language to extract meaningful information, identify patterns, and draw insights. This analysis encompasses various aspects of speech, including acoustic features, linguistic content, intonation, rhythm, and more. It is utilized across different fields for diverse purposes, such as speech recognition, speaker identification, language identification, speech pathology, and emotion recognition. Concerning emotion recognition, speech analysis is part of affective computing. Also indicated as emotion AI, it is a field within AI and human-computer interaction that focuses on the study and development of systems and devices that can recognize, interpret, process, and simulate human emotions. The primary goal is to create more natural and intuitive interactions between humans and machines by enabling computers to understand and respond to the emotional states of users. Facial movements and expressions and physiological signals are also used to detect emotions. For instance, some AUs are more involved in positive (e.g., AU6 and AU12 in smiling) motions whereas other AUs) are mostly associated with negative emotions, such as AU4 in fear or sadness [114].

In the context of speech emotion recognition, the focus is on analyzing the acoustic features of the voice, such as pitch, tone, rhythm, and intensity, to identify patterns associated with different emotional states. There are multiple applications. For example, Beyond Verbal is a technology tool (with an application) for emotion recognition using vocal intonation [115].

In the 1970s, Paul Ekman introduced the discrete model of emotions, which includes six fundamental emotions: anger, disgust, fear, joy, sadness, and surprise (the Big Six) [116] (Fig. 3.5).

An alternative viewpoint was presented by Russell and Mehrabian, who proposed a dimensional approach showing that emotions can be situated along three primary dimensions: valence (positive to negative), arousal (engaged to not engaged), and dominance (level of control over emotional states) [117]. The pleasure-arousal-dominance (PAD) model, also known as the Valence-Arousal-Dominance (VAD) model, was later introduced [118]. This model provides three independent dimensions: pleasure (valence), which ranges from unhappiness to happiness and expresses the pleasant or unpleasant feeling about something; arousal,

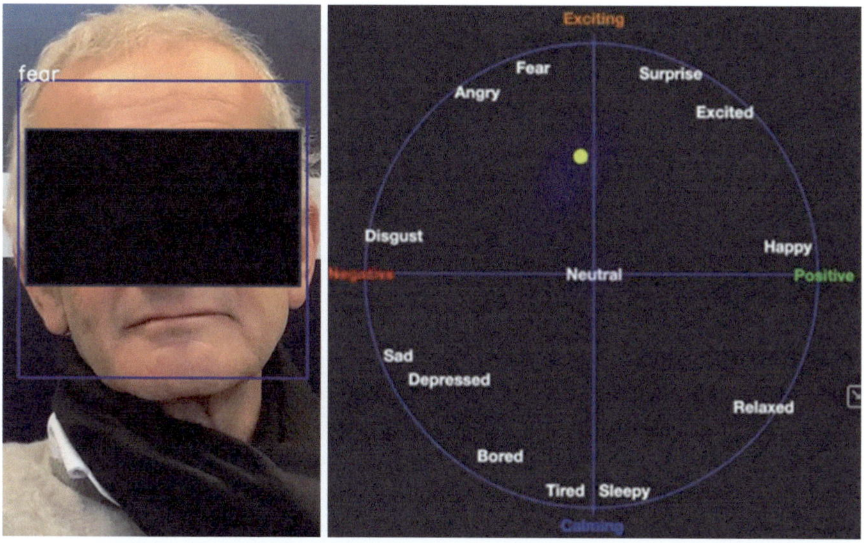

Fig. 3.5 Real-time sentiment analysis in a cancer patient. The analysis was conducted using a Multilayer Perceptron Classifier, comprising five dense layers. The input layer contains 181 nodes corresponding to prosodic features extracted from the audio clip of each image. The three hidden layers have 300, 200, and 100 nodes, respectively. The output layer represents seven emotional states: disgust, joy, fear, anger, surprise, sadness, and neutral. We utilized the rectified linear unit (ReLU) activation function and the adaptive moment estimation (Adam) algorithm for weight optimization. The Softmax function was applied to the output layer to generate the probability distribution across the seven emotional states. Cross-entropy loss guided the training process. Clinical Trial registration: NCT04726228 https://www.clinicaltrials.gov/study/NCT04726228?cond=NCT04726228&rank=1

the level of affective activation ranging from sleep to excitement; and dominance, reflecting the level of control over the emotional state, from submissive to dominant.

Importantly, NLP represents a pivotal advancement in language analysis for pain assessment. Combining computer science, AI, and linguistics, NLP focuses on tasks like classification, annotation, and prediction. NLP applications range from language-enabled virtual assistants to chatbots. The various phases of NLP include tokenization, morphological and lexical analysis, syntactic analysis, generation of parse trees, named entity recognition, semantic analysis, and speech analysis.

AI has a burgeoning role in speech analysis, particularly in sentiment analysis, an NLP technique used to determine and extract subjective information from spoken language. The goal is to understand the sentiment, attitude, or opinion expressed, whether it is positive, negative, or neutral. Sentiment analysis often employs machine learning models to automatically classify sentiment, trained on labeled datasets where human annotators categorize the sentiment of each text sample.

Common algorithms used include SVM, Naive Bayes, and DL models like recurrent architectures and CNNs. Additionally, lexicon-based approaches use dictionaries associating words with sentiment scores to determine the sentiment of text by aggregating individual word scores.

Given these features, language analysis can be effectively implemented for APA. In particular, language analysis for pain assessment involves two key processes: language feature extraction and classification. The verbal taxonomy of pain, particularly the pain descriptor system (PDS), which includes 24 descriptors and 8 subcategories, serves as a foundational classification framework. This system supports diverse investigations, such as survey analyses on pain-related issues [119]. However, pain-related analysis poses unique challenges due to the subjective and multifaceted nature of pain. To address these challenges, specialized lexicons, such as the one validated by Chaturvedi et al. [120] with 382 terms for selecting pain-related elements from electronic health records, have been developed.

The field is dynamic, with continual improvements in NLP algorithms such as Word2Vec and GloVe, which analyze linguistic corpora datasets to understand representative words, sentences, and phrases. A systematic review evaluating NLP applications in low back pain and spinal disease highlighted the versatility of rule-based and ML approaches, underscoring ongoing advancements in leveraging NLP for pain-related studies [121]. The new LLMs offer remarkable research opportunities. The evolutionary progress of these models is so rapid that it is challenging to enumerate them all [122]. As a result, they started being used in pain research as well. For example, Silva-Filho et al. [123] investigated how ChatGPT, might be used in conjunction with transcranial direct current stimulation to manage chronic pain. Additionally, Kunze et al. [124] conducted a proof-of-concept analysis demonstrating the suitability and effectiveness of GPT-4 in triaging, synthesizing differential diagnoses, and generating treatment plans for common knee pain presentations.

Other behavioral strategies have been explored. For instance, Walsh et al. [125] examined the relationship between body posture and pain. In their experiments, 16 actors posed in various body postures to depict pain, and 20 observers selected the most effective images. After validation, a set of 144 images was established. They developed a stimulus set and, during validation, identified "head averted," "gaze downward," and "forward body lean" as common pain-related postures performed by actors. Based on these findings, it was suggested that reduced head motion and altered postures could serve as indicators of pain. In line with these findings, Werner et al. [112] discovered that head movements and postures often orient downward or toward the pain location. Probably, there is also a gender difference in the decoding of pain-related body postures [126, 127]. Finally, head poses can be combined with AUs analysis [112].

A summary of APA strategies is given in Table 3.2.

Table 3.2 Automatic Pain Assessment Methods and AI Applications. ^Can include biosignal-based analyses (accelerometry) and head poses. Abbreviations: AUs, Action Units; NLP, Natural Language Processing; EDA, Electrodermal Activity; EEG, Electroencephalography; ECG, Electrocardiography; EMG, Electromyography; sEMG, surface EMG; PPG, Photoplethysmography; fMRI, functional Magnetic Resonance Imaging; fNIRS, functional Near-infrared Spectroscopy

Category	Method	Description	Examples	Advantages	Challenges	Ref.
Behavioral-based approaches	Facial expressions analysis	Analyzes facial movements and expressions to detect pain	AI-based facial recognition models from AUs or head poses	Non-invasive, captures immediate emotional response	Model building from AUs or complex preprocessing for head pose	[99–112]
	Linguistic analysis	Studies the language and tone used by patients to describe pain	NLP algorithms applied to patient reports and clinical notes	Provides insights into subjective pain experience	Subjectivity in language, requires high-level expertise and large datasets for training	[118–123]
	Non-verbal^ physical indicators	Monitors body movements and posture changes associated with pain	Motion capture systems, accelerometers, and video analysis	Can be used continuously; non-invasive	Requires complex setup, influenced by individual movement patterns	[111, 124–126]
Neurophysiology-based pain detection methods	EDA	Measures skin conductance, which changes with sweat gland activity related to pain and stress	Platform with EDA sensors	Sensitive to autonomic nervous system changes	Susceptible to environmental factors like humidity and temperature	[56–58]

(continued)

Table 3.2 (continued)

Category	Method	Description	Examples	Advantages	Challenges	Ref.
	EEG	Records electrical activity of the brain to detect pain-related patterns	EEG headsets, brain wave analysis software	Direct measurement of brain activity, real-time data	Requires extensive signal processing, can be affected by noise and artifacts	[37–52]
	ECG	Monitors heart rate and its variability as indicators of pain	Wearable ECG monitors, heart rate variability (HRV) analysis tools	Provides continuous monitoring, well-established method	Influenced by other factors like physical activity and emotions	[53–55, 71, 72]
	EMG/sEMG	Measure and record the electrical activity of muscles	Can be used to investigate behavior (movements)	Less invasive or not invasive (sEMG)	The link between muscle tension and pain should be dissected	[59–62]
	Pupillometry	Pupillary unrest under ambient light (PUAL) and the variation coefficient of pupillary diameter	High-resolution cameras.	Non-invasive	Require further investigations.	[67]
	PPG	Uses light-based technology to detect blood volume changes in the microvascular bed of tissue	PPG sensors in wearable devices, smartwatches	Non-invasive, can be integrated into everyday devices	Affected by motion artifacts, requires calibration for accurate readings	[63–66]
	fMRI	Measures brain activity by detecting changes in blood flow	fMRI scanners, neuroimaging software	High spatial resolution provides detailed brain activity maps	Expensive, requires specialized facilities and equipment, not suitable for continuous monitoring	[37–52]

Category	Method	Description	Examples	Advantages	Challenges	Ref.
	fNIRS	Real-time feedback on cerebral oxygenation and blood flow	Pain signatures	Faster acquisition of data. Portable equipment	Superficial measures of cortical brain function	[86–94]
	Thermography	Uses infrared cameras to detect changes in skin temperature related to pain	Infrared thermography cameras, thermal imaging software	Non-invasive; provides continuous monitoring	Affected by ambient temperature, requires specialized equipment	[95–97]
	Eye tracking	Monitors eye movements and as indicators of pain	Video-based eye tracking systems	Non-invasive, provides real-time data	Requires specialized equipment, influenced by lighting conditions	[99]

3.6 Challenges and Perspectives

As previously explained, key aspects include selecting the optimal dataset, feature engineering, and the entire processing phase. A frequently insurmountable challenge is defining the outcome "pain" in terms of binary or multiclass classification (e.g., mild, moderate, severe pain) or discrete terms. Most models use binary classification because adding more classes often leads to significant challenges in maintaining model efficiency. For example, one of the most widely used tools for facial pain recognition, OpenFace©, might be effective at distinguishing between pain and no pain, but its accuracy in classifying pain intensity is questionable [107].

One of the most challenging aspects of research in this field is choosing the various elements to include in the study framework. This is likely the most effective strategy for addressing a multidimensional problem such as pain. When addressing emotions, for instance, our experience of the world, including both the perception and arousal of emotions, is inherently multimodal. Consequently, effective affective computing methods must assess the relative importance of individual unimodal inputs and the interactions between various multimodal sources [128]. Thus, for APA, combining behavioral and physiological data holds promise for developing more accurate predictive models, acknowledging pain as a multidimensional experience influenced by physiological, psychological, and emotional factors.

Another crucial aspect is integrating objective physiological parameters measured through APA with the subjective insights obtained from self-reports. This step is essential to recognize the significance of each feature under consideration and carefully harmonize them to draw comprehensive conclusions that genuinely encompass the intricacies of pain experiences. In recent research on cancer pain, we conducted a multidimensional statistical approach (i.e., sensitivity analysis, multiple factorial analysis, and hierarchical clustering on principal components) based on demographic, clinical, and pain-related variables, as well as EDA and ECG signals. As main result, we failed to find a correlation between pain perception and objective variables of APA [129]. Future research, involving larger and more diverse participant samples, rigorous validation of biosignal-based approaches, and controlled experimental designs, holds the potential to yield a deeper understanding of pain assessment and management strategies [130].

A key aspect to address is the definition of the research outcome. The complexity of the model can differ significantly based on how the outcome is framed. If the outcome is approached as a classification problem, where the task is to distinguish between pain and no pain, the model needs to be designed to effectively differentiate between these two states. This might involve focusing on binary classification techniques and ensuring that the model can effectively recognize and categorize the presence or absence of pain. On the other hand, if the research aims to assess pain intensity (scoring), the model must accurately gauge varying levels of pain intensity rather than simply distinguishing between pain and no pain. Such an approach typically requires methods capable of dealing with continuous variables, and it may involve more complex data processing and interpretation strategies [103, 112].

Concerning multimodal strategies, recently, Peng et al. [131] implemented fNIRS and physiological monitoring for real-time data analysis to evaluate the intraoperative analgesic status of patients, categorizing their pain levels as either "pain alert" or "pain off." Other researchers developed a multimodal method for pain detection, learning features from both videos and biomedical signals. They performed dynamic facial expression analysis, focusing on head poses, and analyzed dynamic biomedical signals from EDA, ECG, and EMG to create a multidimensional representation of pain. For data fusion, five types of features were extracted from each sample: distance-based dynamic features, dynamic head pose features, dynamic biomedical features, and dynamic facial texture features (including dynamic appearance gradient features and GME features). The random forest classifier was employed for both binary and multiclass pain classification. To integrate the five types of descriptors, both feature-level fusion and decision-level fusion were used. Feature-level fusion involves combining features from different modalities (here video and biomedical signals) into a single feature vector before classification. In this approach, features extracted from each modality are concatenated into a long feature vector. This combined feature set is then used as input to an ML classifier. Decision-level fusion combines the outputs of multiple classifiers, each trained on different features or modalities, to make a final decision.

Each classifier produces a decision (here a pain level prediction), and these decisions are then combined, often using methods like majority voting, weighted averaging, or other ensemble techniques, to produce a final classification. The authors obtained accuracies of 85% for feature-level fusion and 86% for decision-level fusion, surpassing the results of single-modality approaches. Notably, biomedical signals were found to be particularly significant in the fusion model [108].

From a fascinating perspective, the implementation of fusion engine strategies could develop a unique vector that considers all different behavioral modalities (text, video, and audio). Such a vector should be composed of selecting only the relevant information across these modalities, and this goal could be achieved by using self-attention techniques. Nevertheless, the fusion of embeddings is highly complex, requiring vector-type data for each dimension. An alternative may involve using a vector database, such as leveraging Milvus, for the three dimensions (video, audio, text) related to pain. For video embedding, several strategies can be used. The open-source pre-trained 3D RESNET model can be easily utilized. An "*N*" hyperparameter is chosen, where *N* identifies the number of frames to process for the video associated with the phrase. If the video has more than *N* frames, exactly *N* frames are taken, evenly distributed. If the video has fewer than *N* frames, additional padding frames are added as needed to reach *N* [132].

Additionally, Bidirectional Encoder Representations from Transformers (BERT) can be adopted for text. It is a state-of-the-art pre-trained natural language processing model developed by Google. BERT typically generates word embeddings in a high-dimensional space, often 768 dimensions. Notably, this transformer architecture allows for efficient parallel processing and captures long-range dependencies in the data. It produces contextualized word embeddings, meaning that the representation of a word can vary depending on its context within a sentence. Finally, for audio embedding extraction, Wav2Vec2 can be used. It is a validated framework for self-supervised learning of speech representations [133]. This approach ensures a robust and comprehensive analysis of pain through the integration of multiple data types, enhancing the accuracy and depth of pain assessment models (Fig. 3.6).

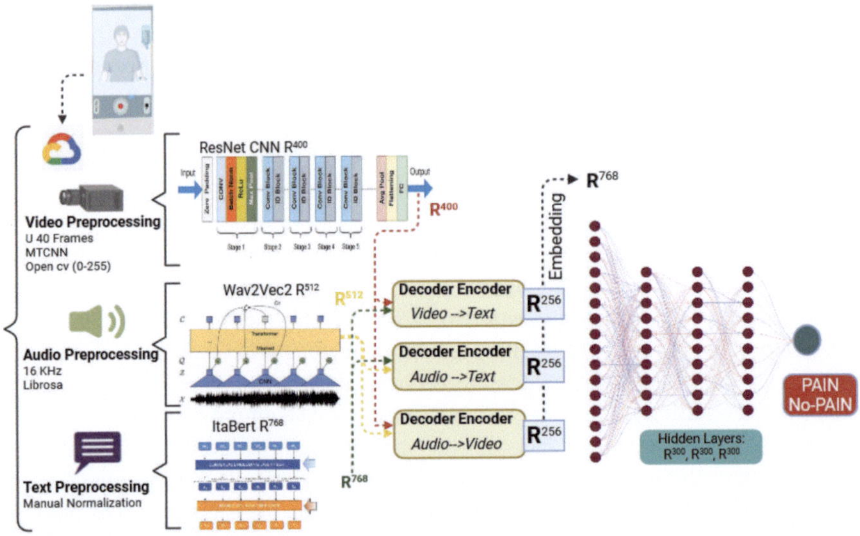

Fig. 3.6 Proposed integrated research framework. A sophisticated approach for automatic pain assessment, utilizing advanced AI techniques to integrate video, audio, and text data. The use of deep learning models like ResNet, Wav2Vec2, and ItaBERT, along with feature translation and integration, showcases the potential for highly accurate and reliable pain detection in clinical settings. In this framework, video recordings are the primary input. Up to 40 frames are extracted (e.g., by using the open-source tool OpenCV) and processed through multi-task cascaded convolutional networks (MTCNN) for face detection. Pixel values are normalized to the 0–255 range to standardize the input for further processing. The audio component is sampled at 16 kHz. Using the Librosa library, relevant features are extracted from the audio signal, preparing it for subsequent analysis. For text preprocessing, textual data, such as transcripts or annotations associated with the video, undergoes manual normalization to ensure consistency and quality, which is crucial for accurate feature extraction. Concerning feature extraction, a Convolutional Neural Network (CNN) based on the ResNet architecture extracts 400-dimensional features (R^400) from the video frames. This network captures critical visual information relevant to pain assessment (video features). A transformer-based model, Wav2Vec2, is utilized to process the audio signal, producing a 512-dimensional feature vector (R^512). This model is designed to capture nuanced auditory cues (Audio Features). Finally, a transformer-based model extracts 768-dimensional features (R^768) from the textual data (Text Features). This model encodes semantic and contextual information from the text, contributing to a comprehensive analysis. Subsequently, modal interaction and feature translation involve three decoder-encoder modules: video-to-text for translating video features into a 256-dimensional textual representation; audio-to-text for translating audio features into a 256-dimensional textual representation; audio-to-video to convert audio features into a 256-dimensional visual representation. The individual features from the video, audio, and text modalities are integrated into a unified 768-dimensional embedding (feature embedding). Three fully connected hidden layers, each with 300 dimensions (R^300), further process the combined embedding. These layers refine the feature representation, enhancing the model's ability to discern complex patterns indicative of pain. The final output layer classifies the processed features into two categories: PAIN or No PAIN

References

1. Raja SN, Carr DB, Cohen M, Finnerup NB, Flor H, Gibson S, Keefe FJ, Mogil JS, Ringkamp M, Sluka KA, Song XJ, Stevens B, Sullivan MD, Tutelman PR, Ushida T, Vader K. The revised International Association for the Study of Pain definition of pain: concepts, challenges, and compromises. Pain. 2020;161:1976–82. https://doi.org/10.1097/j.pain.0000000000001939.
2. Bonezzi C, Fornasari D, Cricelli C, Magni A, Ventriglia G. Not all pain is created equal: basic definitions and diagnostic work-up. Pain Ther. 2020;9:1–15. https://doi.org/10.1007/s40122-020-00217-w.
3. Costigan M, Scholz J, Woolf CJ. Neuropathic pain: a maladaptive response of the nervous system to damage. Annu Rev Neurosci. 2009;32:1–32. https://doi.org/10.1146/annurev.neuro.051508.135531.
4. Cascella M, Muzio MR, Monaco F, Nocerino D, Ottaiano A, Perri F, Innamorato MA. Pathophysiology of nociception and rare genetic disorders with increased pain threshold or pain insensitivity. Pathophysiology. 2022;29(3):435–52. https://doi.org/10.3390/pathophysiology29030035.
5. Cohen SP, Vase L, Hooten WM. Chronic pain: an update on burden, best practices, and new advances. Lancet. 2021;397:2082–97. https://doi.org/10.1016/S0140-6736(21)00393-7.
6. Cascella M, Bimonte S, Saettini F, Muzio MR. The challenge of pain assessment in children with cognitive disabilities: features and clinical applicability of different observational tools. J Paediatr Child Health. 2019;55(2):129–35. https://doi.org/10.1111/jpc.14230.
7. Caraceni A, Shkodra M. Cancer pain assessment and classification. Cancers (Basel). 2019;11(4):510. https://doi.org/10.3390/cancers11040510.
8. Poquet N, Lin C. The brief pain inventory (BPI). J Physiother. 2016;62(1):52. https://doi.org/10.1016/j.jphys.2015.07.001.
9. Ngamkham S, Vincent C, Finnegan L, Holden JE, Wang ZJ, Wilkie DJ. The McGill pain questionnaire as a multidimensional measure in people with cancer: an integrative review. Pain Manag Nurs. 2012;13(1):27–51. https://doi.org/10.1016/j.pmn.2010.12.003.
10. Melzack R. The short-form McGill pain questionnaire. Pain. 1987;30(2):191–7. https://doi.org/10.1016/0304-3959(87)91074-8.
11. Katz J, Melzack R. Measurement of pain. Surg Clin North Am. 1999;79(2):231–52. https://doi.org/10.1016/s0039-6109(05)70381-9.
12. Schmitt JS, Abbott JH. Patient global ratings of change did not adequately reflect change over time: a clinical cohort study. Phys The. 2014;94:534–42. https://doi.org/10.2522/ptj.20130162.
13. Apkarian AV, Hashmi JA, Baliki MN. Pain and the brain: specificity and plasticity of the brain in clinical chronic pain. Pain. 2011;152(Suppl. 3):S49–64. https://doi.org/10.1016/j.pain.2010.11.010.
14. Emmert K, Breimhorst M, Bauermann T, Birklein F, Van De Ville D, Haller S, et al. Comparison of anterior cingulate vs. insular cortex as targets for real-time fMRI regulation during pain stimulation. Front Behav Neurosci. 2014;8:350. https://doi.org/10.3389/fnbeh.2014.00350.
15. Friebel U, Eickhoff SB, Lotze M. Coordinate-based meta-analysis of experimentally induced and chronic persistent neuropathic pain. NeuroImage. 2011;58(4):1070–80.
16. Geha P, Waxman SG. Pain perception: multiple matrices or one? JAMA Neurol. 2016;73(6):628–30. https://doi.org/10.1001/jamaneurol.2016.0757.
17. Mouraux A, Diukova A, Lee MC, Wise RG, Iannetti GD. A multisensory investigation of the functional significance of the "pain matrix". NeuroImage. 2011;54(3):2237–49.
18. Iannetti GD, Hughes NP, Lee MC, Mouraux A. Determinants of laser-evoked EEG responses: pain perception or stimulus saliency? J Neurophysiol. 2008;100(2):815–28. https://doi.org/10.1152/jn.00097.2008.
19. Salomons TV, Iannetti GD, Liang M, Wood JN. The "pain matrix" in pain-free individuals. JAMA Neurol. 2016;73(6):755–6. https://doi.org/10.1001/jamaneurol.2016.0653.

20. Clarke S, Rogers R, Wanigasekera V, Fardo F, Pia H, Nochi Z, Macian N, Leray V, Finnerup NB, Pickering G, Mouraux A, Truini A, Treede RD, Garcia-Larrea L, Tracey I. Systematic review and co-ordinate based meta-analysis to summarize the utilization of functional brain imaging in conjunction with human models of peripheral and central sensitization. Eur J Pain. 2024;28:1069. https://doi.org/10.1002/ejp.2251.
21. Menon V. 20 years of the default mode network: a review and synthesis. Neuron. 2023;111:2469–87. https://doi.org/10.1016/j.neuron.2023.04.023.
22. Heukamp NJ, Moliadze V, Mišić M, Usai K, Löffler M, Flor H, Nees F. Beyond the chronic pain stage: default mode network perturbation depends on years lived with back pain. Pain. 2024;166:160. https://doi.org/10.1097/j.pain.0000000000003335.
23. Alshelh Z, Marciszewski KK, Akhter R, Di Pietro F, Mills EP, Vickers ER, Peck CC, Murray GM, Henderson LA. Disruption of default mode network dynamics in acute and chronic pain states. Neuroimage Clin. 2017;17:222–31. https://doi.org/10.1016/j.nicl.2017.10.019.
24. Johansson E, Xiong HY, Polli A, Coppieters I, Nijs J. Towards a real-life understanding of the altered functional behaviour of the default mode and salience network in chronic pain: are people with chronic pain overthinking the meaning of their pain? J Clin Med. 2024;13(6):1645. https://doi.org/10.3390/jcm13061645.
25. Fox MD, Snyder AZ, Vincent JL, Corbetta M, Van Essen DC, Raichle ME. The human brain is intrinsically organized into dynamic, anticorrelated functional networks. Proc Natl Acad Sci USA. 2005;102:9673–8. https://doi.org/10.1073/pnas.0504136102.
26. De Ridder D, Vanneste S, Smith M, Adhia D. Pain and the triple network model. Front Neurol. 2022;13:757241. https://doi.org/10.3389/fneur.2022.757241.
27. Cascella M, Schiavo D, Cuomo A, Ottaiano A, Perri F, Patrone R, Migliarelli S, Bignami EG, Vittori A, Cutugno F. Artificial intelligence for automatic pain assessment: research methods and perspectives. Pain Res Manag. 2023;2023:6018736. https://doi.org/10.1155/2023/6018736.
28. Cascella M, Schiavo D, Grizzuti M, Romano MC, Coluccia S, Bimonte S, Cuomo A. Implementation of a hybrid care model for telemedicine-based cancer pain management at the Cancer Center of Naples, Italy: a cohort study. In Vivo. 2023;37(1):385–92. https://doi.org/10.21873/invivo.13090.
29. Cascella M, Capuozzo M, Ferrara F, Ottaiano A, Perri F, Sabbatino F, Conti V, Santoriello V, Ponsiglione AM, Romano M, Amato F, Piazza O. Two-year opioid prescription trends in local sanitary agency Naples 3 south, Campania region, Italy. Descriptive analyses and AI-based translational perspectives. Transl Med UniSa. 2024;26(1):1–14. https://doi.org/10.37825/2239-9747.1047.
30. Biancuzzi H, Dal Mas F, Brescia V, Campostrini S, Cascella M, Cuomo A, Cobianchi L, Dorken-Gallastegi A, Gebran A, Kaafarani HM, Marinangeli F, Massaro M, Renne A, Scaioli G, Bednarova R, Vittori A, Miceli L. Opioid misuse: a review of the Main issues, challenges, and strategies. Int J Environ Res Public Health. 2022;19(18):11754. https://doi.org/10.3390/ijerph191811754.
31. Puntmann VO. How-to guide on biomarkers: biomarker definitions, validation and applications with examples from cardiovascular disease. Postgrad Med J. 2009;85(1008):538–45. https://doi.org/10.1136/pgmj.2008.073759.
32. Grouper H, Löffler M, Flor H, Eisenberg E, Pud D. Increased functional connectivity between limbic brain areas in healthy individuals with high versus low sensitivity to cold pain: a resting state fMRI study. PLoS One. 2022;17(4):e0267170. https://doi.org/10.1371/journal.pone.0267170.
33. Ploner M, Lee MC, Wiech K, Bingel U, Tracey I, Romo R. Prestimulus functional connectivity determines pain perception in humans. Proc Natl Acad Sci USA. 2010;107(1):355. https://www.jstor.org/stable/40536278. https://doi.org/10.1073/pnas.0906186106.
34. Martucci KT, Mackey SC. Neuroimaging of pain. Anesthesiology. 2018;128:1241–54.
35. Duerden EG, Albanese MC. Localization of pain-related brain activation: a meta-analysis of neuroimaging data. Hum Brain Mapp. 2013;34(1):109–49.

36. Lin W, Zhou F, Yu L, Wan L, Yuan H, Wang K, Svensson P. Quantitative sensory testing of periauricular skin in healthy adults. Sci Rep. 2020;10(1):3728. https://doi.org/10.1038/s41598-020-60724-w.
37. Levitt J, Saab CY. What does a pain 'biomarker' mean and can a machine be taught to measure pain? Neurosci Lett. 2019;702:40–3. https://doi.org/10.1016/j.neulet.2018.11.038.
38. Zis P, Liampas A, Artemiadis A, Tsalamandris G, Neophytou P, Unwin Z, Kimiskidis VK, Hadjigeorgiou GM, Varrassi G, Zhao Y, Sarrigiannis PG. EEG recordings as biomarkers of pain perception: where do we stand and where to go? Pain Ther. 2022;11(2):369–80. https://doi.org/10.1007/s40122-022-00372-2.
39. Misra G, Wang WE, Archer DB, Roy A, Coombes SA. Automated classification of pain perception using high-density electroencephalography data. J Neurophysiol. 2017;117(2):786–95. https://doi.org/10.1152/jn.00650.2016.
40. dos Pinheiro ESS, de Queirós FC, Montoya P, et al. Electroencephalographic patterns in chronic pain: a systematic review of the literature. PLoS One. 2016;11(2):e0149085.
41. Simis M, Pacheco-Barrios K, Uygur-Kucukseymen E, Castelo-Branco L, Battistella LR, Fregni F. Specific electroencephalographic signatures for pain and descending pain inhibitory system in spinal cord injury. Pain Med. 2022;23(5):955–64. https://doi.org/10.1093/pm/pnab124.
42. Vuckovic A, Hasan MA, Fraser M, Conway BA, Nasseroleslami B, Allan DB. Dynamic oscillatory signatures of central neuropathic pain in spinal cord injury. J Pain. 2014;15(6):645–55.
43. Savignac C, Ocay DD, Mahdid Y, Blain-Moraes S, Ferland CE. Clinical use of electroencephalography in the assessment of acute thermal pain: a narrative review based on articles from 2009 to 2019. Clin EEG Neurosci. 2022;53(2):124–32. https://doi.org/10.1177/15500594211026280.
44. Nir RR, Sinai A, Raz E, Sprecher E, Yarnitsky D. Pain assessment by continuous EEG: association between subjective perception of tonic pain and peak frequency of alpha oscillations during stimulation and at rest. Brain Res. 2010;1344:77–86. https://doi.org/10.1016/j.brainres.2010.05.004.
45. Chen D, Zhang H, Kavitha PT. Scalp EEG-based pain detection using convolutional neural network. IEEE Trans Neural Syst Rehabil Eng. 2022;30:274–85. https://doi.org/10.1109/TNSRE.2022.3147673.
46. Levitt J, Edhi MM, Thorpe RV. Pain phenotypes classified by machine learning using electroencephalography features. NeuroImage. 2020;223:117256. https://doi.org/10.1016/j.neuroimage.2020.117256.117256.
47. Nezam T, Boostani R, Abootalebi V, Rastegar K. A novel classification strategy to distinguish five levels of pain using the EEG signal features. IEEE Trans Affect Comput. 2021;12(1):131–40. https://doi.org/10.1109/TAFFC.2018.2851236.
48. Elsayed M, Sim KS, Tan SC. A novel approach to objectively quantify the subjective perception of pain through electroencephalogram signal analysis. IEEE Access. 2020;8:199920–30. https://doi.org/10.1109/ACCESS.2020.3032153.
49. Feng L, Li H, Cui H, Xie X, Xu S, Hu Y. Low back pain assessment based on alpha oscillation changes in spontaneous electroencephalogram (EEG). Neural Plast. 2021;2021:8537437. https://doi.org/10.1155/2021/8537437.8537437.
50. Vijayakumar V, Case M, Shirinpour S, He B. Quantifying and characterizing tonic thermal pain across subjects from EEG data using random forest models. IEEE Trans Biomed Eng. 2017;64:2988–96. https://doi.org/10.1109/TBME.2017.2756870.
51. Vuckovic A, Gallardo VJF, Jarjees M, Fraser M, Purcell M. Prediction of central neuropathic pain in spinal cord injury based on EEG classifier. Clin Neurophysiol. 2018;129(8):1605–17. https://doi.org/10.1016/j.clinph.2018.04.750.
52. Wei M, Liao Y, Liu J. EEG beta-band spectral entropy can predict the effect of drug treatment on pain in patients with herpes zoster. J Clin Neurophysiol. 2022;39(2):166–73. https://doi.org/10.1097/WNP.0000000000000758.
53. Kim Y, Yoon HY, Kwon IK, Youn I, Han S. Heart rate variability as a potential indicator of cancer pain in a mouse model of peritoneal metastasis. Sensors. 2022;22:2152.

54. Tiwari R, Kumar R, Malik S, Raj T, Kumar P. Analysis of heart rate variability and implication of different factors on heart rate variability. Curr Cardiol Rev. 2021;17:e160721189770.
55. Jean WH, Sutikno P, Fan SZ, Abbod MF, Shieh JS. Comparison of deep learning algorithms in predicting expert assessments of pain scores during surgical operations using analgesia nociception index. Sensors (Basel). 2022;22(15):5496. https://doi.org/10.3390/s22155496.
56. Critchley HD. Electrodermal responses: what happens in the brain. Neuroscientist. 2002;8(2):132–42. https://doi.org/10.1177/107385840200800209.
57. Moscato S, Cortelli P, Chiari L. Physiological responses to pain in cancer patients: a systematic review. Comput Methods Prog Biomed. 2022;217:106682.
58. Egan D, Brennan S, Barrett J, Qiao Y, Timmerer C, Murray N. An evaluation of heart rate and electrodermal activity as an objective QoE evaluation method for immersive virtual reality environments. In: 2016 eighth international conference on quality of multimedia experience (QoMEX). IEEE; 2016. p. 1–6.
59. Qin R, Meng H, Li M. Continuous pain related behavior recognition from muscle activity and body movements. In: 12th international conference on natural computation, fuzzy systems and knowledge discovery (ICNC-FSKD), Changsha, China, vol. 2016; 2016. p. 1710–5. https://doi.org/10.1109/FSKD.2016.7603435.
60. Bongiorno G, Miceli L. EMG surface analysis in short track in line speed skating athletes: the curve after the straight. J Sports Med Phys Fitness. 2023;63(8):906–7. https://doi.org/10.23736/S0022-4707.23.15010-9.
61. Dawes TR, Eden-Green B, Rosten C, Giles J, Governo R, Marcelline F, Nduka C. Objectively measuring pain using facial expression: is the technology finally ready? Pain Manag. 2018;8(2):105–13. https://doi.org/10.2217/pmt-2017-0049.
62. Mieronkoski R, Syrjälä E, Jiang M, Rahmani A, Pahikkala T, Liljeberg P, Salanterä S. Developing a pain intensity prediction model using facial expression: a feasibility study with electromyography. PLoS One. 2020;15(7):e0235545. https://doi.org/10.1371/journal.pone.0235545.
63. Moscato S, Lo Giudice S, Massaro G, Chiari L. Wrist photoplethysmography signal quality assessment for reliable heart rate estimate and morphological analysis. Sensors. 2022;22(15):5831. https://doi.org/10.3390/s22155831.
64. Cao R, Aqajari SAH, Kasaeyan Naeini E, Rahmani AM. Objective pain assessment using wrist-based PPG signals: a respiratory rate based method. In: Proceedings of the annual international conference of the IEEE engineering in medicine and biology society; 2021. p. 1164–7.
65. Kasaeyan Naeini E, Jiang M, Syrjälä E, et al. Prospective study evaluating a pain assessment tool in a postoperative environment: protocol for algorithm testing and enhancement. JMIR Res Protoc. 2009;9(7):e17783. https://doi.org/10.2196/17783.e1778352.
66. Thiam P, Schwenker F. Multi-modal data fusion for pain intensity assessment and classification. In: Proceedings of the 2017 Seventh international conference on image processing theory, tools and applications (IPTA); 2017. p. 1–653.
67. Kyle BN, McNeil DW. Autonomic arousal and experimentally induced pain: a critical review of the literature. Pain Res Manag. 2014;19(3):159–67.
68. Morrill MI, Mace RA, Greenberg J, Lin A, Choi KW, Vranceanu AM. An exploratory analysis of accelerometer-measured physical activity and emotional functioning in patients with chronic pain. J Acad Consult Liaison Psychiatry. 2021;62(2):234–42. https://doi.org/10.1016/j.psym.2020.10.006.
69. Abdollahi M, Ashouri S, Abedi M, Azadeh-Fard N, Parnianpour M, Khalaf K, et al. Using a motion sensor to categorize nonspecific low back pain patients: a machine learning approach. Sensors (Basel). 2020;20(12):3600.
70. Maczák B, Vadai G, Dér A, Szendi I, Gingl Z. Detailed analysis and comparison of different activity metrics. PLoS One. 2021;16:e0261718.
71. Pan J, Tompkins WJ. A real-time QRS detection algorithm. IEEE Trans Biomed Eng. 1985;32:230–6.

72. Moeyersons J, Amoni M, Van Huffel S, Willems R, Varon C. R-DECO: an open-source Matlab based graphical user interface for the detection and correction of R-peaks. PeerJ Comput Sci. 2019;5:e226.
73. Thiam P, Hihn H, Braun DA, Kestler HA, Schwenker F. Multi-modal pain intensity assessment based on physiological signals: a deep learning perspective. Front Physiol. 2021;12:1.
74. Liikkanen S, Mäkinen M, Huttunen T, Sarapohja T, Stenfors C, Eccleston C. Body movement as a biomarker for use in chronic pain rehabilitation: an embedded analysis of an RCT of a virtual reality solution for adults with chronic pain. Front Pain Res (Lausanne). 2022;3:1085791. https://doi.org/10.3389/fpain.2022.1085791.
75. Bach DR, Friston KJ, Dolan RJ. An improved algorithm for model-based analysis of evoked skin conductance responses. Biol Psychol. 2013;94:490–7.
76. Benedek M, Kaernbach C. A continuous measure of phasic electrodermal activity. J Neurosci Methods. 2010;190:80–91.
77. Greco A, Valenza G, Lanata A, Scilingo EP, Cit L. cvxEDA: a convex optimization approach to electrodermal activity processing. IEEE Trans Biomed Eng. 2016;63:797–804.
78. Taylor S, Jaques N, Chen W, Fedor S, Sano A, Picard R. Automatic identification of artifacts in electrodermal activity data. In: 2015 37th annual international conference of the IEEE Engineering in Medicine and Biology Society (EMBC). IEEE; 2015. p. 1934–7.
79. Chow MS, Wu SL, Webb SE, Gluskin K, Yew DT. Functional magnetic resonance imaging and the brain: a brief review. World J Radiol. 2017;9(1):5–9. https://doi.org/10.4329/wjr.v9.i1.5.
80. Iwabuchi SJ, Xing Y, Cottam WJ, Drabek MM, Tadjibaev A, Fernandes GS, Petersen KK, Arendt-Nielsen L, Graven-Nielsen T, Valdes AM, Zhang W, Doherty M, Walsh D, Auer DP. Brain perfusion patterns are altered in chronic knee pain: a spatial covariance analysis of arterial spin labelling MRI. Pain. 2020;161(6):1255–63. https://doi.org/10.1097/j.pain.0000000000001829.
81. Shokouhi M, Davis KD, Moulin DE, Morley-Forster P, Nielson WR, Bureau Y, St Lawrence K. Basal ganglia perfusion in fibromyalgia is related to pain disability and disease impact: an arterial spin labeling study. Clin J Pain. 2016;32(6):495–505. https://doi.org/10.1097/AJP.0000000000000295.
82. Liu J, Hao Y, Du M, Wang X, Zhang J, Manor B, Jiang X, Fang W, Wang D. Quantitative cerebral blood flow mapping and functional connectivity of postherpetic neuralgia pain: a perfusion fMRI study. Pain. 2013;154(1):110–8. https://doi.org/10.1016/j.pain.2012.09.016.
83. Howard MA, Krause K, Khawaja N, Massat N, Zelaya F, Schumann G, Huggins JP, Vennart W, Williams SC, Renton TF. Beyond patient reported pain: perfusion magnetic resonance imaging demonstrates reproducible cerebral representation of ongoing post-surgical pain. PLoS One. 2011;6(2):e17096. https://doi.org/10.1371/journal.pone.0017096.
84. Duong TQ, et al. Microvascular BOLD contribution at 4 and 7 T in the human brain: gradient-echo and spin-echo fMRI with suppression of blood effects. Magn Reson Med. 2003;49:1019–27.
85. Warbrick T. Simultaneous EEG-fMRI: what have we learned and what does the future hold? Sensors (Basel). 2022;22(6):2262. https://doi.org/10.3390/s22062262.
86. Ferrari M, Quaresima V. A brief review on the history of human functional near-infrared spectroscopy (fNIRS) development and fields of application. NeuroImage. 2012;63(2):921–35. https://doi.org/10.1016/j.neuroimage.2012.03.049.S1053-8119(12)00330-8.
87. Naseer N, Hong K. fNIRS-based brain-computer interfaces: a review. Front Hum Neurosci. 2015;9:3. https://doi.org/10.3389/fnhum.2015.00003.
88. Altınkaynak M, Yeşilbaş D, Batbat T, Güven A, Uğurgöl E, Demirci E, İzzetoğlu M, Dolu N. Multimodal analysis of cortical activation in young male adults with internet gaming disorder: a resting state EEG-fNIRS study. J Psychiatr Res. 2024;177:368–77. https://doi.org/10.1016/j.jpsychires.2024.07.019.
89. Ortega-Martinez A, Rogers D, Anderson J, Farzam P, Gao Y, Zimmermann B, Yücel MA, Boas DA. How much do time-domain functional near-infrared spectroscopy (fNIRS)

moments improve estimation of brain activity over traditional fNIRS? Neurophotonics. 2023;10(1):013504. https://doi.org/10.1117/1.NPh.10.1.013504.
90. Racek AJ, Hu X, Nascimento TD, Bender MC, Khatib L, Chiego D, Holland GR, Bauer P, McDonald N, Ellwood RP, DaSilva AF. Different brain responses to pain and its expectation in the dental chair. J Dent Res. 2015;94(7):998–1003. https://doi.org/10.1177/0022034515581642.0022034515581642.
91. Hu X, Racek AJ, Bellile E, Nascimento TD, Bender MC, Toback RL, Burnett D, Khatib L, McMahan R, Kovelman I, Ellwood RP, DaSilva AF. Brain functional changes before, during, and after clinical pain. J Dent Res. 2018;97(5):523–9. https://doi.org/10.1177/0022034517750136.
92. Sugawara AT, De Pretto LR, Simis M, Fregni F, Battistella LR. Primary motor area activity in phantom limb imagery of traumatic unilateral lower limb amputees with phantom limb pain. Adv Rehab Sci Pract. 2024;13:27536351241261023. https://doi.org/10.1177/27536351241261023.
93. Yan T, Liang M, Peng J, Yu Q, Li Y, Yang J, Zhang S, Wang C. Cortical mechanisms underlying effects of repetitive peripheral magnetic stimulation on dynamic and static postural control in patients with chronic non-specific low Back pain: a double-blind randomized clinical trial. Pain Ther. 2024;13(4):953–70. https://doi.org/10.1007/s40122-024-00613-6.
94. Feng Y, Xia Y, Fan B, Li S, Zhang Z, Fang J. Global trends and performances of infrared imaging technology studies on acupuncture: a bibliometric analysis. Front Neurosci. 2024;18:1387752. https://doi.org/10.3389/fnins.2024.1387752.
95. Ohashi Y, Uchida I. Applying dynamic thermography in the diagnosis of breast cancer. IEEE Eng Med Biol Mag. 2000;19(3):42–51. https://doi.org/10.1109/51.844379.
96. Fernández-Cuevas I, Marins JCB, Lastras JA, et al. Classification of factors influencing the use of infrared thermography in humans: a review. Infrared Physics Tech. 2015;71:28–55.
97. Suzuki T, Oishi N, Fukuyama H. Simultaneous infrared thermal imaging and laser speckle imaging of brain temperature and cerebral blood flow in rats. J Biomed Optics. 2019;24:1–11.
98. Liu H, Zhu Z, Jin X, Huang P. The diagnostic accuracy of infrared thermography in lumbosacral radicular pain: a prospective study. J Orthop Surg Res. 2024;19(1):409. https://doi.org/10.1186/s13018-024-04910-w.
99. Schmidt K, Gamer M, Forkmann K, Bingel U. Pain affects visual orientation: an eye-tracking study. J Pain. 2018;19(2):35–145. https://doi.org/10.1016/j.jpain.2017.09.005.
100. Chambers CT, Mogil JS. Ontogeny and phylogeny of facial expression of pain. Pain. 2015;156(5):798–9. https://doi.org/10.1097/j.pain.0000000000000133.
101. Hassan T, Seus D, Wollenberg J, Weitz K, Kunz M, Lautenbacher S, et al. Automatic detection of pain from facial expressions: a survey. IEEE Trans Pattern Anal Mach Intell. 2021;43(6):1815–31. https://doi.org/10.1109/TPAMI.2019.2958341.
102. Werner P, Lopez-Martinez D, Walter A-HA, Gruss S, Picard R. Automatic recognition methods supporting pain assessment: a survey. IEEE Trans Affect Comput. 2019;13:530–52. https://doi.org/10.1109/TAFFC.2019.2946774.
103. Ekman P, Friesen WV. Facial action coding system: a technique for the measurement of facial movement. Edina, MN: Consulting Psychologists Press; 1978.
104. Prkachin KM, Solomon PE. The structure, reliability and validity of pain expression: evidence from patients with shoulder pain. Pain. 2008;139(2):267–74. https://doi.org/10.1016/j.pain.2008.04.010.
105. Lucey P, Cohn JF, Prkachin KM. Painful data: the UNBC-McMaster shoulder pain expression archive database. In: Automatic Face & Gesture Recognition and workshops (FG 2011) IEEE international conference on IEEE. IEEE; 2011. p. 57–64.
106. Cascella M, Vitale VN, Mariani F, Iuorio M, Cutugno F. Development of a binary classifier model from extended facial codes toward video-based pain recognition in cancer patients. Scand J Pain. 2023;23(4):638–45. https://doi.org/10.1515/sjpain-2023-0011.
107. Gomutbutra P, Kittisares A, Sanguansri A, Choosri N, Sawaddiruk P, Fakfum P, Lerttrakarnnon P, Saralamba S. Classification of elderly pain severity from automated video clip facial action

unit analysis: a study from a Thai data repository. Front Artif Intell. 2022;5:942248. https://doi.org/10.3389/frai.2022.942248.
108. Zhi R, Yu J. Multi-modal fusion based automatic pain assessment. 2019 IEEE 8th joint international information technology and artificial intelligence conference (ITAIC), Chongqing, China, vol. 2019. IEEE; 2019. p. 1378–82. https://doi.org/10.1109/ITAIC.2019.8785727.
109. Nanni L, Lumini A, Brahnam S. Local binary patterns variants as texture descriptors for medical image analysis. Artif Intell Med. 2010;49(2):117–25.
110. Rodriguez P, Cucurull G, Gonzalez J. Deep pain: exploiting long short-term memory networks for facial expression classification. IEEE Trans Cyber. 2017;99:1–11.
111. Lu G, Li X, Li H. Research on recognition for facial expression of pain in neonates. Acta Opt Sin. 2008;28(11):2109–14.
112. Werner P, Al-Hamadi A, Limbrecht-Ecklundt K, Walter S, Gruss S, Traue HC. Automatic pain assessment with facial activity descriptors. IEEE Trans Affect Comput. 2016;1:1–14. https://doi.org/10.1109/TAFFC.2016.2537327.
113. Tian Y. Artificial intelligence image recognition method based on convolutional neural network algorithm. IEEE Access. 2020;8:125731–44. https://doi.org/10.1109/ACCESS.2020.3006097.
114. Luneski A, Konstantinidis E, Bamidis PD. Affective medicine. A review of affective computing efforts in medical informatics. Methods Inf Med. 2010;49(3):207–18. https://doi.org/10.3414/ME0617.
115. Beyond Verbal. https://www.predictiveanalyticstoday.com/beyond-verbal/. Accessed 25 July 2024.
116. Ekman P, Sorenson ER, Friesen WV. Pan-cultural elements in facial displays of emotions. Science. 1969;164:86–8.
117. Russell JA, Mehrabian A. Evidence for a three-factor theory of emotions. J Re Personal. 1977;11:273–94.
118. Mehrabian A. Pleasure-arousal-dominance: a general framework for describing and measuring individual differences in temperament. Curr Psychol. 1996;14:261–92.
119. Fernandez E, Vargas R, Mahometa M, Ramamurthy S, Boyle GJ. Descriptors of pain sensation: a dual hierarchical model of latent structure. J Pain. 2012;13(6):532–6. https://doi.org/10.1016/j.jpain.2012.02.006.
120. Chaturvedi J, Mascio A, Velupillai SU, Roberts A. Development of a lexicon for pain. Front Digit Health. 2021;3:778305. https://doi.org/10.3389/fdgth.2021.778305.778305.
121. Bacco L, Russo F, Ambrosio L, D'Antoni F, Vollero L, Vadalà G, Dell'Orletta F, Merone M, Papalia R, Denaro V. Natural language processing in low back pain and spine diseases: a systematic review. Front Surg. 2022;9:957085. https://doi.org/10.3389/fsurg.2022.957085.
122. Cascella M, Semeraro F, Montomoli J, Bellini V, Piazza O, Bignami E. The breakthrough of large language models release for medical applications: 1-year timeline and perspectives. J Med Syst. 2024;48(1):22. https://doi.org/10.1007/s10916-024-02045-3.
123. Silva-Filho E, Pegado R. ChatGPT and transcranial direct current stimulation for chronic pain. Innov Clin Neurosci. 2024;21(61–62):1–3.
124. Kunze KN, Varady NH, Mazzucco M, Lu AZ, Chahla J, Martin RK, Ranawat AS, Pearle AD, Williams RJ 3rd. The large language model ChatGPT-4 demonstrates excellent triage capabilities and diagnostic performance for patients presenting with various causes of knee pain. Arthroscopy. 2024;S0749–8063(24):00456. https://doi.org/10.1016/j.arthro.2024.06.021.
125. Walsh J, Eccleston C, Keogh E. Pain communication through body posture: the development and validation of a stimulus set. Pain. 2014;155(11):2282–90. https://doi.org/10.1016/j.pain.2014.08.019.
126. Werner P, Al-Hamadi A, Limbrecht-Ecklundt K, Walter S, Traue HC. Head movements and postures as pain behavior. PLoS One. 2018;13(2):e0192767. https://doi.org/10.1371/journal.pone.0192767.
127. Walsh J, Eccleston C, Keogh E. Sex differences in the decoding of pain-related body postures. Eur J Pain. 2017;21(10):1668–77. https://doi.org/10.1002/ejp.1072.

128. Cortinas-Lorenzo K, Lacey G. Toward explainable affective computing: a review. IEEE Trans Neural Netw Learn Syst. 2023;35:13101. https://doi.org/10.1109/TNNLS.2023.3270027.
129. Cascella M, Di Gennaro P, Crispo A, Vittori A, Petrucci E, Sciorio F, Marinangeli F, Ponsiglione AM, Romano M, Ovetta C, Ottaiano A, Sabbatino F, Perri F, Piazza O, Coluccia S. Advancing the integration of biosignal-based automated pain assessment methods into a comprehensive model for addressing cancer pain. BMC Palliat Care. 2024;23(1):198. https://doi.org/10.1186/s12904-024-01526-z.
130. Cascella M, Vitale VN, D'Antò M, Cuomo A, Amato F, Romano M, Ponsiglione AM. Exploring biosignals for quantitative pain assessment in cancer patients: a proof of concept. Electronics. 2023;12(17):3716. https://doi.org/10.3390/electronics12173716.
131. Peng K, Karunakaran KD, Green S, Borsook D. Machines, mathematics, and modules: the potential to provide real-time metrics for pain under anesthesia. Neurophotonics. 2024;11(1):010701. https://doi.org/10.1117/1.NPh.11.1.010701.
132. 3D RESNET model. https://pytorch.org/hub/facebookresearch_pytorchvideo_resnet/. Accessed 2 Oct 2023.
133. Baevski A, Zhou H, Mohamed A, Auli M. wav2vec 2.0: a framework for self-supervised learning of speech representations. arXiv:2006.11477. 2006.

4 Clinical Applications of AI in Pain Medicine

The integration of AI in pain medicine is rooted in broader advances in digital health and biomedical informatics. Early applications focused on data management and simple predictive models. Pioneering studies, for example, demonstrated the feasibility of using AI and computational strategies to help in the diagnosis of pain conditions, such as low back [1] and abdominal pain [2]. With the advent of big data and advanced ML techniques in the 2010s, AI's role expanded to more sophisticated tasks, such as image analysis and more complex predictive analytics heralding a new era of precision pain medicine, in different clinical scenarios [3]. Since ML algorithms and DL can analyze complex datasets to identify patterns and make predictions, in pain medicine, AI can be implemented for different aims. For example, in the field of computer-aided diagnosis (CAD), attempts have been made to enhance the diagnostic accuracy of pain [4, 5], predict treatment outcomes [6], and personalize pain management strategies [7]. Furthermore, in terms of generative AI, NLP enables the extraction of valuable insights from clinical notes and patient reports and can be used to develop dedicated chatbots [8]. Again, automated tools, such as smartphone applications and wearable devices, have been developed to offer real-time monitoring and analysis of pain-related data. These advanced modalities can allow the analysis of diverse data sources, including self-reported pain scales, facial expressions, and both behavioral and physiological signals [9]. Methods for objective pain assessment, such as those based on physiological signals or behavioral phenomena, are addressed in a dedicated chapter of the book.

4.1 Computer-Aided Diagnosis

AI-driven diagnostic processes can be particularly valuable in complex cases where pain etiology is multifactorial and not easily discernible [10]. The idea is that multimodal approaches could be suitable to provide a more accurate and comprehensive assessment of pain compared to relying solely on subjective self-reports.

© The Author(s), under exclusive license to Springer Nature Switzerland AG 2024
M. Cascella, *Exploring AI in Pain Research and Management*, https://doi.org/10.1007/978-3-031-78833-8_4

Consequently, different CAD strategies have been proposed to assist clinicians in making more accurate diagnoses.

Studies have demonstrated varying levels of accuracy in pain intensity assessments, with overall promising results for AI-driven pain evaluation. For instance, Fontaine et al. [11] found that their DL model (ResNet-18 convolutional neural network) developed to detect and classify 2810 facial expressions of 1189 patients, evaluated before and after surgery, had a sensitivity of 89.7% for detecting pain, 77.5% for severe pain, and an accuracy of 53% in estimating pain intensity. Conversely, Bargshady et al. [12] employed a three-stream hybrid deep neural network (i.e., ensemble deep learning model) to train a pain database. They reported an accuracy of 89 and an AUC ROC of 94% for shoulder pain estimation. Similarly, Hosseini et al. [13] used a DL model featuring a transfer learning technique, where a pre-trained CNN model was adopted by replacing the dense upper layers, and the model was tuned using painful facial to identify seven-level thresholds from facial expression images. Additionally, Barua et al. [14] implemented the deep network DarkNet19 pre-trained on ImageNet1K and achieved a high accuracy of 95% in estimating self-induced shoulder pain. These studies focused on the facial expression for pain recognition. Other strategies have been proposed, particularly for low back pain. For example, Abdollahi et al. [15] conducted an observational study using an inertial measurement unit (IMU), a motion tracking system that measures a body's specific force, angular rate, and sometimes the magnetic field surrounding the body, to collect kinematic data. The aim was to create a kinematic sensor-based ML model that could classify nonspecific lower back pain (NSLBP) patients into high and low-risk groups. The study involved 94 patients with NSLBP and utilized a support vector machine (SVM) and an ANN (multi-layer perceptron, MLP) for classification. The findings indicated that kinematic data could classify patients with 75% accuracy using SVM and 60% accuracy using MLP. On the same clinical issue, Staartjes et al. [16] performed a prospective study to determine the efficacy of the Five Repetition Sit to Stand Test (5R-STS) as a diagnostic tool for low back pain and leg pain. This study involved 292 patients and utilized a fuzzy rule-based system. The results demonstrated a high accuracy of approximately 96% when using 5R-STS results combined with ML to classify patients as having lumbar disk herniation, lumbar spinal stenosis, or NSLBP. Furthermore, Liew et al. [17] conducted an observational study using motion capture with electromyography assessments on participants during lifting and exercise activities. They aimed to evaluate the use of ML models in classifying healthy controls and low back pain subgroups using functional physiological signals. The study involved 49 participants, categorized into healthy controls ($n = 16$), low back pain in remission ($n = 16$), and current low back pain ($n = 17$). Their ML technology achieved high accuracy in classifying low back pain status directly, with an AUC of 90.4% for control vs. current pain, 91.2% for control vs. pain in remission, and 96.7% for chronic pain in remission vs. current low back pain.

CAD strategies can be implemented for complex pain conditions. Fibromyalgia (FM) patients exhibit altered cognitive and emotional processing, often allocating attention preferentially to pain-related information. This attention bias toward pain cues can impair cognitive functions such as inhibitory control, which in turn affects patients' ability to manage and express emotions. Sentiment analysis using large language models (LLMs) can offer valuable insights by detecting nuances in pain expression. In a study involving 40 FM patients and 40 non-FM chronic pain controls, researchers analyzed transcribed responses to questions about pain and sleep using the LLM Mistral-7B-Instruct-v0.2. They employed two approaches: one using prompt engineering to target FM-associated language nuances ("prompt-engineered") and another without this targeting ('ablated'). The prompt-engineered approach demonstrated superior performance with an accuracy of 0.87, precision of 0.92, recall of 0.84, specificity of 0.82, and an AUC ROC of 0.86 for distinguishing FM. In comparison, the ablated approach had an accuracy of 0.76, precision of 0.75, recall of 0.77, specificity of 0.75, and an AUC ROC of 0.76. The improved accuracy of the prompt-engineered approach was statistically significant (McNemar's test $p < 0.001$). This proof-of-concept study suggests that LLM-driven sentiment analysis, particularly with prompt engineering, may aid in diagnosing FM by detecting subtle differences in pain expression [5].

In another investigation, Lapitov et al. [18] used neuroimaging data alone (MRI diffusion tensor and T1-weighted imaging) to identify subclasses of neuropathic facial pain. Their ML models using random forest (RF) and logistic regression distinguished classical trigeminal neuralgia from health controls with up to 95% accuracy. Interestingly, the classifiers identified selected gray and white matter-based predictive metrics. Fascinating approaches are focused on the application of fNIRS for pain detection. Peng et al. [19] tested an ML model to provide real-time metrics for pain under general anesthesia.

4.2 Integration of AI Within a Comprehensive Multimodal Model

AI can enhance traditional diagnostic methods by providing additional layers of analysis and insight. Therefore, the research also focused on a comprehensive approach with AI models developed for analyzing complex physiological and clinical information. In this context, Lee et al. [20] developed an experimental study to create ML models that could objectively classify a patient's pain level using neuroimaging and autonomic metrics. The study involved 53 patients with chronic lower back pain and used SVM and support vector regression (SVR) as the AI technologies. The classification of pain levels within individual patients achieved an accuracy of 92.45%, with an AUC ROC of 0.97. The regression model developed to predict pain in new patients demonstrated a significant result, with a correlation coefficient (r) of 0.63.

Interestingly, other authors developed a database of different biosignals including electromyography, skin conductance level, and electrocardiography. They carried out an experimental study aimed at creating an ML pain recognition system that could objectively categorize pain levels based on biopotential data. The study involved 85 participants who were subjected to controlled levels of painful heat stimuli (baseline, pain threshold, two intermediate thresholds, and pain tolerance threshold). A total of 159 features were extracted from the mathematical groupings. Using SVM, the ML model achieved high classification rates with 91% accuracy for baseline versus pain tolerance threshold and 79% accuracy for baseline versus pain threshold [21].

The diagnosis of chronic pain must necessarily consider the plethora of conditions that collectively structure the pain experience. Soin et al. [22] conducted a pilot study to implement an ML algorithm for diagnosing spinal conditions in chronic pain settings. The authors examined whether AI via ML algorithms could analyze specific data points to predict diagnoses related to spinal pain in a prospective, observational pilot study involving 246 patients. Patients completed a Google form on an iPad with 85 data points, including demographic information and pain-related details, which a decision tree ML model then processed. The predictions were compared with practitioner-assigned diagnoses, revealing a 72% accuracy rate. As the authors stated, while the study demonstrated promise for AI-augmented decision-making in diagnosing spinal conditions, further research to refine these approaches and explore categorizing patients based on biopsychosocial factors and data from patient-owned devices is needed.

Proper cancer pain diagnosis and management is often challenging. In a recent study, we employed a comprehensive statistical approach, including sensitivity analysis, multiple factorial analysis, and hierarchical clustering on principal components. This analysis incorporated demographic, clinical, and pain-related variables, along with electrodermal activity and electrocardiogram signals. Multifactorial analysis revealed correlations between pain intensity, pain type, Eastern Cooperative Oncology Group (ECOG) performance status, opioid usage, and the presence of metastases. Clustering analysis identified three distinct patient groups based on pain characteristics, treatments, and ECOG. Additionally, multivariable regression analysis demonstrated associations between pain intensity, breakthrough cancer pain (a typical cancer pain phenomenon) [23], and opioid dosages [24].

On the other hand, the combination of data from different sources may be challenging for the risk of bias. Therefore, despite advancements, extensive validation from clinical studies is needed before AI-based pain recognition tools can receive widespread approval and practical implementation [23].

4.3 Predictive Models for Disease Progression

Predictive models utilize multisource patient data to forecast the likelihood of pain and disease progression. Knee osteoarthritis is a common painful disease with important impairment of the quality of life and functionality. In a proof-of-concept study with a sample size of 216 patients suffering from knee osteoarthritis followed in a long follow-up, Lin et al. [25] developed and tested a nomogram that implemented MRI scans and patient characteristics to predict improvement in the disease. In particular, they adopted the least absolute shrinkage and selection operator (LASSO) regression for feature selection and multivariate logistic regression for nomogram creation. The nomogram demonstrated good performance in both the training and test sets, with AUC ROC values of 0.79 and 0.83 for predicting a 20% improvement in pain symptoms over 2 years.

Furthermore, Guan et al. [26] conducted a retrospective AI-driven analysis on a dataset with features related to 9348 knees from 4674 subjects with or at risk for knee osteoarthritis. Deep learning models trained with knee radiographs demonstrated superior diagnostic performance, with AUC ROC values of 0.807 and 0.77, compared to traditional models that used only demographic, clinical, and radiographic risk factors (AUC of 0.69).

Additionally, other researchers developed a model for predicting knee pain in middle-aged and elderly individuals. They implemented different ML algorithms including logistic regression, RF, and extreme data boosting, and found that logistic regression exhibited the greatest accuracy in predicting knee pain, achieving an AUC of 0.71 [27].

Since chronic pain is a complex biopsychosocial phenomenon, understanding the connection between emotional states, pain, and bodily sensations can offer important data on the disease progression. On these bases, Goldstein et al. [28] used a mobile platform (cliexa-EASE) for collecting data on pain and emotional states in patients with chronic back pain. Given these data, they developed two models for predicting future pain, with or without pain-related features. Both models were implemented to predict pain 2 weeks later. The results showed that the predictive accuracies were 65% and 72% concerning the two models created.

4.4 AI-Based Pain Treatments

Different strategies have been proposed for implementing AI-based models for pain treatment. For example, the most suitable pathway for spinal cord stimulation is a key topic. Patient selection, trial duration and modality, potential trial avoidance, and treatment planning are a matter of debate. The use of predictive analytics could offer paramount information to guide the decision-making process. In this scenario, Andres et al. [29] implemented ML and imaging biomarkers, based on the idea that chronic pain is linked to changes in brain structure and function. The process for selecting ideal candidates for spinal cord stimulation therapy involved analyzing functional variables and pain evaluation scores. The study included 24 patients, with 7 classified as responders. Notably, combining clinical variables with significant imaging biomarkers increased diagnostic accuracy in the responders' group from 29% to 96%, indicating a high success rate.

To proceed with the real-world evaluations of AI strategies, the accuracy of the models must reach an acceptable level, generally up to 0.72. This goal is often difficult to obtain. For instance, d'Hollosy et al. [30] used ML algorithms to determine whether patient data could aid in decision-making for low back pain treatment. The dataset included patient-reported data from a spine center via a biopsychosocial questionnaire with 287 input features. The algorithms predicted whether patients needed "Pain Rehabilitation Treatment" or "Pain Surgery Treatment," considering only models with AUC scores above 0.55. The best-performing models, BayesNet and Naive Bayes achieved an AUC score of only 0.67. The authors acknowledged the limitations of using imbalanced data and cost-sensitive learning to reduce false predictions.

Improved efficacy, increasing access, and reducing costs are the main goals of healthcare policies. In a randomized trial, Piette et al. [31] evaluated a cognitive behavioral therapy (CBT) intervention for chronic back pain that used artificial intelligence to adjust treatment based on patient progress feedback. This intervention was compared to standard telephone-based CBT for chronic pain (CBT-CP) in terms of reducing therapist time. The study found that the outcomes of the AI-driven CBT were comparable to those of traditional 45-min telephone sessions, despite requiring less than half the therapist's time. At the 6-month mark, a higher proportion of patients in the AI-CBT-CP group showed significant improvements in physical function and pain intensity. Significantly, they implemented a reinforcement learning strategy as the trial design allocated more patients to the AI-CBT-CP group than to the control group (1.4:1) to enhance the system's learning from patient interactions.

4.5 Diagnosis and Management of Opioid Use Disorders

The opioid crisis is a plague difficult to eradicate. Predictive analytics could offer interesting perspectives. Interestingly, researchers developed an ML algorithm for early detection of opioid use disorder (OUD) using data from a commercial claims database spanning from 2006 to 2018, including ten million medical insurance claims from 55,000 patients. They tested ML's effectiveness in creating a prediction model for early OUD diagnosis, using 436 predictors grouped into demographics, chronic conditions, diagnoses and procedures, medication features, medical costs, and episode counts. The Word2Vec and Gradient Boosting Trees algorithms were used for analysis, yielding a *C*-statistic of 0.959, with sensitivity and specificity of 0.85 and 0.882, respectively. The positive predictive value was 0.362, while the negative predictive value was 0.998. Significant differences were found between positive and negative OUD groups in various factors, including opioid use days, prescription overlaps, and pain-related diagnoses. Their findings suggest that the model potentially reduces the time to diagnose OUD by an average of 14.4 months, reducing morbidity, medical costs, addictions, and mortality. However, the need for replication and further evaluation was emphasized to confirm its usefulness in early OUD diagnosis [32].

Electronic Health Records (EHRs) are increasingly being used to perform different descriptive and predictive analyses. Banks et al. [33] recently utilized the Veterans Administration's EHR data with approximately 28,000 patients diagnosed with OUD, to develop AI models for predicting new OUD diagnoses. They analyzed patient features to determine their predictive value for new OUD diagnoses across two time periods: 2000–2012 and 2013–2021. Three different AI-based techniques were employed including logistic regression, RF, and a deep learning architecture, all achieving an accuracy of over 80% in predicting OUD. Using a RF classifier, they found that opioid prescription features, such as early refills and prescription length, consistently ranked among the top five predictors of new OUD. Additionally, younger age was positively correlated with new OUD, while older age showed an inverse relationship. Age stratification indicated that prior substance abuse and alcohol dependency were more significant predictors of OUD in younger patients. On the contrary, no significant differences were found in the factors associated with new OUD between the two time periods. The authors concluded that opioid prescription characteristics are the most impactful predictors of new OUD both before and after the peak in opioid prescribing rates and that predictive models should be tailored to different age groups.

Unstructured such as the notes for patient admission or other notes can be analyzed via NLP models. Using the freely accessible critical care MIMIC-III database [34] for analyses, researchers utilized structured and unstructured parts of the EHR to develop a deep learning model to predict opioid prescription. The models achieved an F1-score of 0.88 with an AUC ROC of 0.93. Another model dedicated to predicting OUD diagnosis achieved an F1-score of 0.82 with an AUC ROC of 0.94 [35].

Fibromyalgia is often treated with opioids due to limited therapeutic options, but long-term opioid use is linked to several adverse outcomes [36]. Identifying factors associated with prolonged opioid use in this population is crucial for developing targeted interventions. To address this problem, Ramírez Medina et al. [37] conducted a retrospective cohort study using the UK Clinical Research Practice Datalink, focusing on fibromyalgia patients who were new opioid users. They employed logistic regression, a RF model, and Boruta feature selection to identify risk factors for long-term opioid use. Among 28,552 fibromyalgia patients who initiated opioid treatment, 7369 (26%) were long-term users. The findings indicated that a high initial opioid dose, history of self-harm, obesity, high deprivation, substance use disorder, and age are strongly associated with long-term opioid use in fibromyalgia patients.

4.6 Prediction of Treatment Response

Several studies have explored the use of AI to predict patient responses to various treatments. In pain medicine, fibromyalgia is a chapter of great interest. Ichesco et al. [38] conducted a double-blind, placebo-controlled crossover study on 28 fibromyalgia patients to predict pharmacologic responses using functional neuroimaging biomarkers and SVM. They highlighted that connectivity patterns in the posterior cingulate cortex and dorsolateral prefrontal cortex could predict responses to pregabalin or milnacipran with 92% accuracy. Verma et al. [39] performed a retrospective data-driven analysis using data from two previous studies ($n = 377$ and $n = 1040$) to investigate the ability of different ML methods to predict outcomes in patients with low back and nonspecific neck pain. They employed seven regression algorithms and two classifier algorithms, finding that regression methods accurately predicted patient-reported outcomes like pain and ability to work, though classifiers struggled with predicting treatment referrals. Interestingly, Tu et al. [40] ran a randomized single-blind trial with 50 chronic lower back pain patients to determine if ML approaches using functional MRI scans could predict responses to real or sham acupuncture. They found that pretreatment resting-state functional connectivity patterns could predict pain changes with a coefficient of determination of 34% and 29% for real and sham acupuncture, respectively. Yet, Branco et al. [41] evaluated if natural language processing could predict placebo analgesia in patients with chronic pain. In a retrospective validation study involving 116 individuals, the AI model used patient language features to predict placebo responses with an AUC ROC of 0.71. Placebo responders experienced a 30% reduction in pain compared to 3% in non-responders.

Researchers from the University of California, San Francisco implanted intracranial electrodes in the anterior cingulate cortex and orbitofrontal cortex (OFC) of four individuals suffering from refractory neuropathic pain for deep brain stimulation. The participants provided pain metrics via a phone app and ambulatory data were systematically collected. Using machine learning techniques, the researchers were able to accurately predict chronic pain severity scores from neural activity within each individual. The decoding of chronic pain depended on sustained power changes in the OFC, which were distinct from the transient activity patterns observed during acute, evoked pain states in task-based settings [42].

4.7 Real-Time Pain Monitoring and Management

Wearable technology and biosensors can enable continuous monitoring of physiological indicators related to pain, such as heart rate variability, skin conductance, and muscle activity. These devices transmit data to AI systems that analyze patterns and detect pain exacerbations in real time. Furthermore, continuous monitoring facilitates timely interventions and enhances pain control. This approach is a key aspect of telehealth.

Telehealth solutions enhance access to pain management, particularly for patients in remote or underserved areas. Consequently, the utilization of AI-based telemedicine pathways in pain medicine holds significant potential to transform medical service delivery. This synergy between AI technologies and telehealth processes has the potential to revolutionize remote patient care by providing more personalized and effective healthcare services.

Different AI applications have been proposed. Researchers explored the capabilities of a specific deep learning model, a generative adversarial network (GAN), and its potential for enhancing telemedicine approaches to cancer pain management. GAN is an AI framework that consists of two antagonistic architectures: the generator and the discriminator network. This strategy can play a notable role in data-driven analyses by generating new data that closely resembles a given dataset. The authors implemented a structured dataset consisting of demographic and clinical variables from 226 patients and 489 telemedicine visits for cancer pain management. The deep learning model, specifically a conditional GAN, was employed to generate synthetic samples that closely resemble real individuals based on their characteristics. Subsequently, four ML algorithms were used to assess the variables associated with a higher number of remote visits. The generated dataset exhibited a distribution comparable to the reference dataset for all considered variables, including age, number of visits, tumor type, performance status, characteristics of metastasis, opioid dosage, and type of pain. Among the tested algorithms, the RF demonstrated the highest performance in predicting a higher number of remote visits, achieving an accuracy of 0.8 on the test data. The ML simulations indicated that individuals younger than 45 years old and those experiencing breakthrough cancer pain may require an increased number of telemedicine-based clinical evaluations [7].

The same authors conducted other research to develop AI-based care models of telemedicine by modulating remote visits and hospital access according to clinical needs and resource allocation [43]. They also tested ML models on a dataset encompassing multiple demographic, social, clinical, and therapeutic variables to intercept the conditions that can affect the number of teleconsultations. Among the results, in the training set, the accuracy was about 95% and 98% for the ANN and RF, respectively. Nevertheless, the best accuracy on the test set was obtained with RF (70%). Subsequently, they performed simulations and found that young age (<55 years), lung cancer, and occurrence of breakthrough cancer pain can assist predict the number of remote consultations.

4.8 AI in Postoperative Pain Management

AI predicts postoperative pain by analyzing preoperative and intraoperative data. Predictive models can identify patients at risk of severe postoperative pain, guiding analgesic planning and intervention strategies.

In a study, Park et al. [44] aimed to determine if an AI model based on facial expressions could accurately predict significant postoperative pain. They gathered 155 facial expressions from patients who had undergone gastric cancer surgery, focusing on facial action units (AUs), gaze, landmarks, and positions. These features were used to build various ML models to differentiate between significant postoperative pain (NRS ≥7) and less significant pain (NRS <7). Relevant AUs predictive of NRS ≥7 were identified and compared to AUs associated with pain in awake patients. The study found that AU17 (chin raising) and AU20 (lip stretching) were associated with NRS ≥7. Interestingly, AUs typically linked to pain in awake patients did not correlate with postoperative pain. The ML model based on AU17 and AU20 had an AUC ROC of 0.62 for predicting NRS ≥7, which was lower than a model using all AUs (AUC ROC = 0.81). Among the facial features, head position and facial landmarks were better predictors of NRS ≥7, with AUC ROCs ranging from 0.85 to 0.96. The best-performing ML model merged gaze, eye landmarks, head position, and facial landmarks, achieving an AUC ROC of 0.90 in predicting significant postoperative pain. Subsequently, the same authors demonstrated that their model based on facial expressions outperformed different models developed from biosignals (i.e., analgesia nociception index), and vital signs [45].

In another investigation, Ohtman et al. [46] created two AI-driven methods to forecast continuous NRS using heart rate data. The first method leveraged machine learning algorithms including polynomial regression, lasso regression, and ridge regression, whereas the second utilizes an LSTM model. Significantly, the deep learning architecture, which does not depend on conventional interpolation methods, demonstrated superior performance compared to the machine learning interpolation-based approach.

4.9 AI and Pain in Special Populations

Machine learning models analyze behavioral and physiological indicators to assess pain levels and guide treatment, ensuring accurate pain management for different special populations. Infants are unable to self-report their pain, leading to frequent underrecognition and undertreatment. Adequate pain assessment, especially for procedural pain, is critical due to its short- and long-term consequences. On the contrary, inadequate pain management is linked to increased avoidance behaviors and heightened social hypervigilance, and it may induce long-term changes in brain structure, such as alterations in cerebral white matter and subcortical gray matter. These changes can result in a range of behavioral, developmental, and learning difficulties [47]. In this vulnerable population, there has been growing interest in employing machine learning techniques to understand behavioral responses to pain by analyzing facial expressions [48], crying sounds [49], and body movements [50]. Additionally, research indicates that automated systems can effectively detect emotions from physiological responses such as pupil dilation [51], galvanic skin response [52], heart rate variability [53], and cerebral hemodynamic fluctuations [54]. Behavioral and physiological methods are combined in multimodal strategies [55]. Tools have been also developed. For example, the PainChek Infant is a mobile health-based (mHealth) solution that utilizes artificial intelligence to assess pain intensity based on facial expressions. The developers evaluated its accuracy and feasibility by observing infants before, during, and after immunization, and testing its performance at various cutoff scores. PainChek Infant proved effective across multiple feasibility aspects, including interpretability, ease of administration, rapid completion time (3 s), and clinician comprehensibility [56]. Additionally, Carlini et al. [57] implemented a CNN-based architecture on two databases including the UNIFESP dataset [58] and the Classification of Pain Expression (iCOPE) [59]. Subsequently, they developed a mobile application that can detect a neonate's face and classify it as either "pain" or "no pain" with low latency and offline capabilities.

Other researchers tested EGG, an AI-based interactive toy designed to estimate individual pain levels and engage children through an immersive experience using visual, tactile, and audio stimuli [60]. Investigations in this population were carried on by implementing multimodal strategies [61]. Additionally, AI applications address the unique pain management needs of elderly patients, who frequently have multiple comorbidities and complex medication regimens. Predictive models identify optimal pain management strategies, considering factors such as frailty and the risks associated with polypharmacy.

AI also aids in monitoring pain in cognitively impaired elderly individuals. For this purpose, AI tools enhance pain assessment in non-verbal and cognitively impaired patients by analyzing non-verbal cues, physiological signals, and caregiver reports. These tools provide objective pain assessments, ensuring that populations receive appropriate pain management and care [62]. For example, the point-of-care medical device PainChek application can also be used for individuals affected by dementia [63, 64]. In a retrospective study, Atee et al. explored pain-related facial expressions in 3144 individuals with dementia using the Face domain of PainChek®. The study involved 389 assessors from 2 national dementia-specific care programs and 34 aged care homes across Australia, generating a total of 22,194 pain assessments. The researchers analyzed the frequency, distribution, and relationships of facial action units (AUs) with varying pain intensities. They found that AU7 (eyelid tightening) was the most common expression during severe pain, appearing in 48.6% of assessments, followed by AU43 (closing eyes) at 42.9% and AU6 (cheek raising) at 42.1%. AU20 (horizontal mouth stretch) was the strongest predictor of higher pain levels. Eye-related AUs (AU6, AU7, AU43) and brow-related AU (AU4) were more prevalent than mouth-related AUs (e.g., AU20, AU25) at higher pain intensities. The study found no significant differences related to age or gender.

Researchers recorded videos of non-communicative patients during activities such as bed bathing, repositioning, or blood pressure measurement to observe whether these procedures elicited pain behaviors. A research assistant trained in dementia pain assessment was tasked with rating the video clips of both communicative and non-communicative patients using the PAINAD score, which assesses five observational domains of pain behavior: breathing, negative vocalization, facial expression, body language, and consolability [65]. The video clips were then automatically coded using the open-source tool OpenFace©. However, in real-world applications, the models have shown unsatisfactory metrics [66].

4.10 Potential Future Applications and Research Areas

Future research areas include the development of AI models for rare pain conditions, the integration of AI with genomics for precision pain medicine, and the use of AI in pain prevention strategies. Exploring the potential of AI in novel therapeutic approaches, such as neuromodulation and regenerative medicine, will expand its applications in pain management. Consequently, the future of AI in pain medicine envisions a seamless integration of AI technologies into clinical practice. AI will support clinicians in delivering personalized, evidence-based care, enhancing patient outcomes and quality of life.

The preliminary step is the testing of the model in real-world scenarios. In other words, clinical trials involving AI in pain medicine can provide evidence of its efficacy and safety. These trials should evaluate AI's role in various aspects of pain management, from diagnosis to treatment personalization.

One promising development is the creation of advanced wearable pain signaling systems, such as smart socks embedded with fabric sensors. As Korving et al. [67] suggested these systems can be designed to detect biosignal responses (e.g., electrodermal activity), which can indicate pain levels in individuals who have difficulty communicating their pain, such as those with severe and profound intellectual disabilities. Machine learning algorithms can be implemented to classify moments of pain with high accuracy and predict pain based on new data. The authors provided an example of an Internet of Things (IoT) application. This connectivity allows for the seamless transmission of data from wearable devices to centralized databases, enabling real-time monitoring and analysis. IoT-enabled devices can communicate with each other, share data, and trigger alerts for caregivers or medical professionals when pain is detected. This interconnected network ensures that pain-related information (and management) is continuous, responsive, and well-coordinated, improving the overall efficacy of the system.

Concerning AI-based pain management, a scoping review concluded that to improve outcomes in chronic pain management, future research should focus on identifying the underlying mechanisms of pain, optimizing pain management strategies, and enhancing rehabilitation techniques. Additionally, since supervised ML methods are commonly implemented, the research should leverage a broader array of algorithms and computational architectures. Finally, according to the authors, explainable AI could be more used [68].

Notably, AI can leverage gamification processes. Gamification involves seamlessly incorporating gaming elements into contexts that typically aren't associated with traditional games. Mostly centered around app-based solutions, these pathways can be implemented for training in pain medicine, self-monitoring, goal setting, social support, and the instruction of self-care strategies, including stress management [69].

It would also be fascinating to explore the practical applications of extended reality (XR) techniques. XR encompasses various modalities designed for immersive and interactive experiences. What ties these approaches together is their integration of the physical world with digital elements, fundamentally transforming our perception of reality. More specifically, XR is an overarching term that includes virtual reality (VR), augmented reality (AR), and mixed reality (MR), along with any technology that creates computer-generated environments. In brief, VR immerses users in entirely virtual worlds, disconnecting them from their physical surroundings. By using specialized equipment like headsets and sometimes hand controllers, users can navigate and interact within these digital spaces, often experiencing a strong sense of presence in the virtual environment. In contrast, AR overlays digital information onto the real world, blending virtual objects with the physical environment.

This integration enhances the creation of interactive and engaging experiences that seamlessly combine digital and real-world elements. MR merges aspects of both VR and AR, enabling users to interact with virtual objects that appear to coexist with their physical surroundings. This technology is mostly used to alleviate pain for pediatric patients during different medical and surgical procedures [70] as well as for home-based pain management [71]. AI could be valuable for optimizing pathways and integrating extracted data within a multimodal framework. Recently, Bugeja et al. [72] investigated the application of VR distraction therapy combined with conditioning techniques for reducing pain perception in different acute and chronic pain conditions. Participants underwent VR therapy while physiological data were collected, and a conditioning stimulus was delivered via a smartwatch. The authors found a significant reduction in pain levels, with an overall decrease of 42% in pain perception.

Selected applications of AI for pain medicine and key metrics of the developed models are reported in Table 4.1.

Table 4.1 A summary of clinical applications of AI in pain medicine

Application	Method, setting/aim	Key findings	References
AI for diagnosing pain conditions	ResNet-18 CNN for postoperative pain	Sensitivity: 89.7%, severe pain detection: 77.5%, pain intensity estimation: 53%	[11]
	Ensemble Deep Learning Model	Accuracy: 89%, AUC ROC: 94% for shoulder pain	[12]
	Transfer learning with pre-trained CNN	Identified seven-level pain thresholds from facial expressions	[13]
	DarkNet19 pre-trained on ImageNet1K	Accuracy: 95% for shoulder pain	[14]
	SVM and ANN. Chronic low back pain	Classification accuracy: SVM (75%), ANN (60%) for NSLBP	[15]
	Fuzzy rule-based system. Low and leg pain	Accuracy: 96% using 5R-STS for lumbar conditions	[16]
	Functional data boosting. Low back pain	AUC: 90.4% (control vs. current pain), 91.2% (control vs. pain in remission)	[17]
	LLM. LLM (Mistral-7B-Instruct-v0.2) for sentiment analysis in fibromyalgia	Accuracy: 87%, precision: 92%, recall: 84%, specificity: 82%	[5]

(continued)

Table 4.1 (continued)

Application	Method, setting/aim	Key findings	References
Comprehensive pain assessment	SVM and SVR	Classification accuracy: 92.45%, AUC: 0.97	[20]
	Biosignal-based pain recognition. SVM	Accuracy: 91% (baseline vs. pain tolerance threshold), 79% (baseline vs. pain threshold)	[21]
	Decision tree ML. Spinal conditions	Accuracy: 72%	[22]
	Random forest, logistic regression. Neuropathic facial pain	Accuracy: 95%	[18]
Predicting disease progression	LASSO regression, multivariate logistic regression. Knee osteoarthritis improvement	AUC: 0.79 (training set), 0.83 (test set)	[25]
	Deep learning on knee radiographs	AUC: 0.807, 0.77	[26]
	Predicting knee pain. Logistic regression, random forest, extreme data boosting	Highest accuracy: logistic regression, AUC: 0.71	
	cliexa-EASE mobile platform—chronic pain	Predictive accuracies: 65% and 72%	[28]
AI for pain treatment	ML and imaging biomarkers. Spinal cord stimulation	Diagnostic accuracy increased from 29% to 96% for	[29]
	BayesNet, Naive Bayes. Chronic pain	Best AUC score: 0.67	[30]
Predicting opioid use disorder	Commercial claims database analysis	*C*-statistic: 0.959, sensitivity: 85%, specificity: 88.2%	[32]
	Logistic regression, random forest, deep learning. Opioids prescription	Accuracy: >80%	[33]
	NLP on EHR data (MIMIC-III). OUD diagnosis	F1-score: 0.88 (opioid prescription), 0.82 (OUD)	[34]
	Logistic regression, random forest, Boruta feature selection. Risk factors for long-term opioid use in fibromyalgia	26% long-term opioid users	[37]
Predicting treatment response	Functional neuroimaging biomarkers, SVM. Chronin pain	Accuracy: 92% for pregabalin or milnacipran response	[38]
	Seven regression algorithms, two classifier algorithms	Regression methods predicted outcomes accurately	[39]
	Functional MRI scans. Acupuncture	Prediction accuracy: 34% (real acupuncture), 29% (sham acupuncture)	[41]
	NLP for predicting placebo analgesia	AUC: 0.71	[42]

Table 4.1 (continued)

Application	Method, setting/aim	Key findings	References
AI for real-time monitoring and telemedicine	GAN for telemedicine in cancer pain management	Accuracy: 0.8 (random forest predicting remote visits)	[7]
	ANN, random forest for telemedicine visits	Training accuracy: 95% (ANN), 98% (RF); test accuracy: 70% (RF)	[43]
Predicting postoperative pain	Various models	Enhanced postoperative pain prediction and management	[44, 45]
Pediatric, elderly, non-verbal patients	Various models and medical device applications (e.g., PainChek)	Enhanced pain assessment	[48–66]

References

1. Mathew B, Norris D, Hendry D, Waddell G. Artificial intelligence in the diagnosis of low-back pain and sciatica. Spine (Phila Pa 1976). 1988;13(2):168–72. https://doi.org/10.1097/00007632-198802000-00007.
2. Sturman MF, Perez M. Computer-assisted diagnosis of acute abdominal pain. Compr Ther. 1989;15(2):26–35.
3. Abd-Elsayed A, Robinson CL, Marshall Z, Diwan S, Peters T. Applications of artificial intelligence in pain medicine. Curr Pain Headache Rep. 2024;28(4):229–38. https://doi.org/10.1007/s11916-024-01224-8.
4. Cascella M, Vitale VN, Mariani F, Iuorio M, Cutugno F. Development of a binary classifier model from extended facial codes toward video-based pain recognition in cancer patients. Scand J Pain. 2023;23(4):638–45. https://doi.org/10.1515/sjpain-2023-0011.
5. Venerito V, Iannone F. Large language model-driven sentiment analysis for facilitating fibromyalgia diagnosis. RMD Open. 2024;10(2):e004367. https://doi.org/10.1136/rmdopen-2024-004367.
6. Zhao Z, Zhao M, Yang T, Li J, Qin C, Wang B, Wang L, Li B, Liu J. Identifying significant structural factors associated with knee pain severity in patients with osteoarthritis using machine learning. Sci Rep. 2024;14(1):14705. https://doi.org/10.1038/s41598-024-65613-0.
7. Cascella M, Scarpati G, Bignami EG, Cuomo A, Vittori A, Di Gennaro P, Crispo A, Coluccia S. Utilizing an artificial intelligence framework (conditional generative adversarial network) to enhance telemedicine strategies for cancer pain management. J Anesth Analg Crit Care. 2023;3(1):19. https://doi.org/10.1186/s44158-023-00104-8.
8. Cascella M, Semeraro F, Montomoli J, Bellini V, Piazza O, Bignami E. The breakthrough of large language models release for medical applications: 1-year timeline and perspectives. J Med Syst. 2024;48(1):22. https://doi.org/10.1007/s10916-024-02045-3.
9. Cascella M, Schiavo D, Cuomo A, Ottaiano A, Perri F, Patrone R, Migliarelli S, Bignami EG, Vittori A, Cutugno F. Artificial intelligence for automatic pain assessment: research methods and perspectives. Pain Res Manag. 2023;2023:6018736. https://doi.org/10.1155/2023/6018736.
10. Vallejo-De la Cueva A, Aretxabala-Cortajarena N, Quintano-Rodero A, Rodriguez-Nuñez C, Pelegrin-Gaspar PM, Gil-Garcia ZI, Margüello-Fernandez AA, Aparicio-Cilla L, Parraza-Diez N. Pupillary dilation reflex and behavioural pain scale: study of diagnostic test. Intensive Crit Care Nurs. 2023;74:103332. https://doi.org/10.1016/j.iccn.2022.103332.

11. Fontaine D, Vielzeuf V, Genestier P, Limeux P, Santucci-Sivilotto S, Mory E, Darmon N, Lanteri-Minet M, Mokhtar M, Laine M, Vistoli D, DEFI study group. Artificial intelligence to evaluate postoperative pain based on facial expression recognition. Eur J Pain. 2022;26(6):1282–91. https://doi.org/10.1002/ejp.1948.
12. Bargshady G, Zhou X, Deo RC, Soar J, Whittaker F, Wang H. Ensemble neural network approach detecting pain intensity from facial expressions. Artif Intell Med. 2020;109:101954. https://doi.org/10.1016/j.artmed.2020.101954.
13. Hosseini E, Fang R, Zhang R, Chuah CN, Orooji M, Rafatirad S, Rafatirad S, Homayoun H. Convolution neural network for pain intensity assessment from facial expression. Annu Int Conf IEEE Eng Med Biol Soc. 2022;2022:2697–702. https://doi.org/10.1109/EMBC48229.2022.9871770.
14. Barua PD, Baygin N, Dogan S, Baygin M, Arunkumar N, Fujita H, Tuncer T, Tan RS, Palmer E, Azizan MMB, Kadri NA, Acharya UR. Automated detection of pain levels using deep feature extraction from shutter blinds-based dynamic-sized horizontal patches with facial images. Sci Rep. 2022;12(1):17297. https://doi.org/10.1038/s41598-022-21380-4.
15. Abdollahi M, Ashouri S, Abedi M, Azadeh-Fard N, Parnianpour M, Khalaf K, et al. Using a motion sensor to categorize nonspecific low back pain patients: a machine learning approach. Sensors (Basel). 2020;20(12):3600.
16. Staartjes VE, Quddusi A, Klukowska AM, Schröder ML. Initial classification of low back and leg pain based on objective functional testing: a pilot study of machine learning applied to diagnostics. Eur Spine J. 2020;29(7):1702–8.
17. Liew BXW, Rugamer D, De Nunzio AM, Falla D. Interpretable machine learning models for classifying low back pain status using functional physiological variables. Eur Spine J. 2024;29(8):1845–59.
18. Latypov TH, So MC, Hung PS, Tsai P, Walker MR, Tohyama S, Tawfik M, Rudzicz F, Hodaie M. Brain imaging signatures of neuropathic facial pain derived by artificial intelligence. Sci Rep. 2023;13(1):10699. https://doi.org/10.1038/s41598-023-37034-y.
19. Peng K, Karunakaran KD, Green S, Borsook D. Machines, mathematics, and modules: the potential to provide real-time metrics for pain under anesthesia. Neurophotonics. 2024;11(1):010701. https://doi.org/10.1117/1.NPh.11.1.010701.
20. Lee J, Mawla I, Kim J, Loggia ML, Ortiz A, Jung C, et al. Machine learning-based prediction of clinical pain using multimodal neuroimaging and autonomic metrics. Pain. 2019;160(3):550–60.
21. Gruss S, Treister R, Werner P, Traue HC, Crawcour S, Andrade A, et al. Pain intensity recognition rates via biopotential feature patterns with support vector machines. PLoS One. 2019;10(10):e0140330.
22. Soin A, Hirschbeck M, Verdon M, Manchikanti L. A pilot study implementing a machine learning algorithm to use artificial intelligence to diagnose spinal conditions. Pain Physician. 2022;25(2):171–8.
23. Cuomo A, Cascella M, Forte CA, Bimonte S, Esposito G, De Santis S, Cavanna L, Fusco F, Dauri M, Natoli S, Maltoni M, Morabito A, Mediati RD, Lorusso V, Barni S, Porzio G, Mercadante S, Crispo A. Careful breakthrough cancer pain treatment through rapid-onset transmucosal fentanyl improves the quality of life in cancer patients: results from the BEST multicenter study. J Clin Med. 2020;9(4):1003. https://doi.org/10.3390/jcm9041003.
24. Cascella M, Di Gennaro P, Crispo A, Vittori A, Petrucci E, Sciorio F, Marinangeli F, Ponsiglione AM, Romano M, Ovetta C, Ottaiano A, Sabbatino F, Perri F, Piazza O, Coluccia S. Advancing the integration of biosignal-based automated pain assessment methods into a comprehensive model for addressing cancer pain. BMC Palliat Care. 2024;23(1):198. https://doi.org/10.1186/s12904-024-01526-z.
25. Lin T, Peng S, Lu S, Fu S, Zeng D, Li J, et al. Prediction of knee pain improvement over two years for knee osteoarthritis using a dynamic nomogram based on MRI-derived radiomics: a proof-of-concept study. Osteoarthr Cartil. 2023;31(2):267–78.
26. Guan B, Liu F, Mizaian AH, Demehri S, Samsonov A, Guermazi A, et al. Deep learning approach to predict pain progression in knee osteoarthritis. Skeletal Radiol. 2022;51(2):363–73.

27. Liu L, Zhu MM, Cai LL, Zhang X. Predictive models for knee pain in middle-aged and elderly individuals based on machine learning methods. Comput Math Methods Med. 2022;2022:5005195.
28. Goldstein P, Ashar Y, Tesarz J, Kazgan M, Cetin B, Wager TD. Emerging clinical technology: application of machine learning to chronic pain assessments based on emotional body maps. Neurotherapeutics. 2020;17(3):774–83. https://doi.org/10.1007/s13311-020-00886-7.
29. Andres JE, Ten-Esteve A, Harutyunyan A, et al. Predictive clinical decision system using machine learning and imaging biomarkers in patients with neurostimulation therapy: a pilot study. Pain Physician. 2021;24:E1279–90.
30. d'Hollosy W, van Velsen, L, Poel M, et al. Applying machine learning on patient-reported data to model the selection of appropriate treatments for low back pain: a pilot study. In: Proceedings of the 13th international joint conference on biomedical engineering systems and technologies (BIOSTEC 2020); 2020. pp. 117–24.
31. Piette JD, Newman S, Krein SL, Marinec N, Chen J, Williams DA, Edmond SN, Driscoll M, LaChappelle KM, Kerns RD, Maly M, Kim HM, Farris KB, Higgins DM, Buta E, Heapy AA. Patient-centered pain care using artificial intelligence and mobile health tools: a randomized comparative effectiveness trial. JAMA Intern Med. 2022;182(9):975–83. https://doi.org/10.1001/jamainternmed.2022.3178.
32. Segal Z, Radinsky K, Elad G, et al. Development of a machine learning algorithm for early detection of opioid use disorder. Pharmacol Res Perspect. 2020;8:e00669.
33. Banks TJ, Nguyen TD, Uhlmann JK, Nair SS, Scherrer JF. Predicting opioid use disorder before and after the opioid prescribing peak in the United States: a machine learning tool using electronic healthcare records. Health Informatics J. 2023;29(2):14604582231168826. https://doi.org/10.1177/14604582231168826.
34. Johnson AE, Pollard TJ, Shen L, Lehman LW, Feng M, Ghassemi M, Moody B, Szolovits P, Celi LA, Mark RG. MIMIC-III, a freely accessible critical care database. Sci Data. 2016;3:160035. https://doi.org/10.1038/sdata.2016.35.
35. Kashyap A, Callison-Burch C, Boland MR. A deep learning method to detect opioid prescription and opioid use disorder from electronic health records. Int J Med Inform. 2023;171:104979. https://doi.org/10.1016/j.ijmedinf.2022.104979.
36. Biancuzzi H, Dal Mas F, Brescia V, Campostrini S, Cascella M, Cuomo A, Cobianchi L, Dorken-Gallastegi A, Gebran A, Kaafarani HM, Marinangeli F, Massaro M, Renne A, Scaioli G, Bednarova R, Vittori A, Miceli L. Opioid misuse: a review of the main issues, challenges, and strategies. Int J Environ Res Public Health. 2022;19(18):11754. https://doi.org/10.3390/ijerph191811754.
37. Ramírez Medina CR, Feng M, Huang YT, Jenkins DA, Jani M. Machine learning identifies risk factors associated with long-term opioid use in fibromyalgia patients newly initiated on an opioid. RMD Open. 2024;10(2):e004232. https://doi.org/10.1136/rmdopen-2024-004232.
38. Ichesco E, Peltier SJ, Mawla I, Harper DE, Pauer L, Harte SE, et al. Prediction of differential pharmacologic response in chronic pain using functional neuroimaging biomarkers and a support vector machine algorithm: an exploratory study. Arthritis Rheumatol. 2021;73(11):2127–37.
39. Verma D, Jansen D, Bach K, Poel M, Mork PJ, d'Hollosy WON. Exploratory application of machine learning methods on patient reported data in the development of supervised models for predicting outcomes. BMC Med Inform Decis Mak. 2022;22(1):227.
40. Tu Y, Ortiz A, Gollub RL, Cao J, Gerber J, Lang C, et al. Multivariate resting-state functional connectivity predicts responses to real and sham acupuncture treatment in chronic low back pain. Neuroimage Clin. 2019;23:101885.
41. Branco P, Berger S, Abdullah T, Vachon-Presseau E, Cecchi G, Apkarian AV. Predicting placebo analgesia in patients with chronic pain using natural language processing: a preliminary validation study. Pain. 2023;164(5):1078–86.
42. Shirvalkar P, Prosky J, Chin G, Ahmadipour P, Sani OG, Desai M, Schmitgen A, Dawes H, Shanechi MM, Starr PA, Chang EF. First-in-human prediction of chronic pain state using

intracranial neural biomarkers. Nat Neurosci. 2023;26(6):1090–9. https://doi.org/10.1038/s41593-023-01338-z.

43. Cascella M, Schiavo D, Grizzuti M, Romano MC, Coluccia S, Bimonte S, Cuomo A. Implementation of a hybrid care model for telemedicine-based cancer pain management at the Cancer Center of Naples, Italy: a cohort study. In Vivo. 2023;37(1):385–92. https://doi.org/10.21873/invivo.13090.
44. Park I, Park JH, Yoon J, Song IA, Na HS, Ryu JH, Oh AY. Artificial intelligence model predicting postoperative pain using facial expressions: a pilot study. J Clin Monit Comput. 2024;38(2):261–70. https://doi.org/10.1007/s10877-023-01100-7.
45. Park I, Park JH, Yoon J, Na HS, Oh AY, Ryu J, Koo BW. Machine learning model of facial expression outperforms models using analgesia nociception index and vital signs to predict postoperative pain intensity: a pilot study. Korean J Anesthesiol. 2024;77(2):195–204. https://doi.org/10.4097/kja.23583.
46. Othman GB, Yumuk E, Copot D, Ynineb AR, Farbakhsh H, Birs IR, Muresan CI, De Keyser R, Chihi I, Ionescu CM, Neckebroek M. Enhancing pain level assessment in post-surgery patients using artificial intelligence algorithms. In: 2024 European control conference (ECC), Stockholm, Sweden; 2024. pp. 3051–6. https://doi.org/10.23919/ECC64448.2024.10590753.
47. Page GG. Are there long-term consequences of pain in newborn or very young infants? J Perinat Educ. 2004;13(3):10–7.
48. Brahnam S, Chuang C-F, Shih FY, Slack MR. Machine recognition and representation of neonatal facial displays of acute pain. Artif Intell Med. 2006;36(3):211–22.
49. Pal P, Iyer AN, Yantorno RE. Emotion detection from infant facial expressions and cries. In: Proceedings of 2006 IEEE international conference on acoustics speech and signal processing, vol. 2, May 2006. p II.
50. Zamzmi G, Pai C-Y, Goldgof D, Kasturi R, Sun Y, Ashmeade T (2017) Automated pain assessment in neonates. In: Proceedings of the 20th scandinavian conference on image analysis. pp. 350–61.
51. Partala T, Surakka V. Pupil size variation as an indication of affective processing. Int J Hum-Comput Stud. 2003;59(1):185–98.
52. Gruss S, Treister R, Werner P, Traue HC, Crawcour S, Andrade A, Walter S. Pain intensity recognition rates via biopotential feature patterns with support vector machines. PLoS One. 2015;10(10):e0140330. https://doi.org/10.1371/journal.pone.0140330.
53. Walter S, Gruss S, Limbrecht-Ecklundt K, Traue HC, Werner P, Al-Hamadi B, Diniz N, da Silva GM, Andrade AO. Automatic pain quantification using autonomic parameters. Psychol Neurosci. 2014;7:363–80. https://doi.org/10.3922/j.psns.2014.041.
54. Ranger M, Glinas C. Innovating in pain assessment of the critically ill: exploring cerebral near-infrared spectroscopy as a bedside approach. Pain Manage Nurs. 2014;15(2):519–29.
55. Zamzmi G, Kasturi R, Goldgof D, Zhi R, Ashmeade T, Sun Y. A review of automated pain assessment in infants: features, classification tasks, and databases. IEEE Rev Biomed Eng. 2018;11:77–96. https://doi.org/10.1109/RBME.2017.2777907.
56. Hughes JD, Chivers P, Hoti K. The clinical suitability of an artificial intelligence-enabled pain assessment tool for use in infants: feasibility and usability evaluation study. J Med Internet Res. 2023;25:e41992. https://doi.org/10.2196/41992.
57. Carlini LP, Ferreira LA, Coutrin GAS, Varoto VV, Heiderich TM, Balda RCX, Barros MCM, Guinsburg R A convolutional neural network-based mobile application to bedside neonatal pain assessment. In: 34th SIBGRAPI conference on graphics, patterns and images (SIBGRAPI), Gramado, Rio Grande do Sul, Brazil; 2021. pp. 394–401. https://doi.org/10.1109/SIBGRAPI54419.2021.00060.
58. Heiderich TM, Leslie AT, Guinsburg R. Neonatal procedural pain can be assessed by computer software that has good sensitivity and specificity to detect facial movements. Acta Paediatr. 2015;104(2):e63–9. https://doi.org/10.1111/apa.12861.

59. Brahnam S, Chuang CF, Sexton RS, Shih FY. Machine assessment of neonatal facial expressions of acute pain. Decis Support Syst. 2007;43(4):1242–54.
60. Li J, Chen K, Yang L, Mutsaers M, Barakova E. EGG: AI-based interactive design object for managing post-operative pain in children. In: Ferrández Vicente JM, Val Calvo M, Adeli H, editors. Artificial intelligence for neuroscience and emotional systems. IWINAC 2024, Lecture notes in computer science, vol. 14674. Cham: Springer; 2024. https://doi.org/10.1007/978-3-031-61140-7_31.
61. Gholami B, Haddad WM, Tannenbaum AR. Relevance vector machine learning for neonate pain intensity assessment using digital imaging. IEEE Trans Biomed Eng. 2010;57(6):1457–66. https://doi.org/10.1109/TBME.2009.2039214.
62. Smith E, Storch EA, Vahia I, et al. Affective computing for late-life mood and cognitive disorders. Front Psychiatry. 2021;12:782183. https://doi.org/10.3389/fpsyt.2021.782183.782183.
63. Atee M, Hoti K, Hughes JD. Psychometric evaluation of the electronic pain assessment tool: an innovative instrument for individuals with moderate-to-severe dementia. Dement Geriatr Cogn Disord. 2018;44(5–6):256–67.
64. Babicova I, Cross A, Forman D, Hughes J, Hoti K. Evaluation of the psychometric properties of PainChek R in UK aged care residents with advanced dementia. BMC Geriatr. 2021;21(1):337.
65. Warden V, Hurley AC, Volicer L. Development and psychometric evaluation of the pain assessment in advanced dementia (PAINTED) scale. J Am Med Dir Assoc. 2003;4:9–15. https://doi.org/10.1097/01.JAM.0000043422.31640.F7.
66. Gomutbutra P, Kittisares A, Sanguansri A, Choosri N, Sawaddiruk P, Fakfum P, Lerttrakarnnon P, Saralamba S. Classification of elderly pain severity from automated video clip facial action unit analysis: a study from a Thai data repository. Front Artif Intell. 2022;5:942248. https://doi.org/10.3389/frai.2022.942248.
67. Korving H, Li S, Zhou D, Sterkenburg P, Markopoulos P, Barakova E. Development of a pain signaling system using machine learning. In: 2023 IEEE international conference on acoustics, speech, and signal processing workshops (ICASSPW), Rhodes Island, Greece, 2023. pp. 1–5. https://doi.org/10.1109/ICASSPW59220.2023.10193643.
68. Khan MA, Koh RGL, Rashidiani S, Liu T, Tucci V, Kumbhare D, Doyle TE. Cracking the chronic pain code: a scoping review of artificial intelligence in chronic pain research. Artif Intell Med. 2024;151:102849. https://doi.org/10.1016/j.artmed.2024.102849.
69. Cascella M, Cascella A, Monaco F, Shariff MN. Envisioning gamification in anesthesia, pain management, and critical care: basic principles, integration of artificial intelligence, and simulation strategies. J Anesth Analg Crit Care. 2024;3(1):33. https://doi.org/10.1186/s44158-023-00118-2.
70. Jones K, Armstrong M, Luna J, Thakkar RK, Fabia R, Groner JI, Noffsinger D, Ni A, Griffin B, Xiang H. Age and sex differences of virtual reality pain alleviation therapeutic during pediatric burn care: a randomized clinical trial. J Med Ext Real. 2024;1(1):163–73. https://doi.org/10.1089/jmxr.2024.0004.
71. Rumzie M, Figura C. Use of virtual reality therapy (VRT) for home-based pain management, an observational cohort study. J Med Ext Real. 2024;1(1):93–9. https://doi.org/10.1089/jmxr.2023.0006.
72. Bugeja A, Dingli A. Pain management and conditioning through virtual reality and affective computing. In: IEEE international conference on bioinformatics and biomedicine (BIBM), Istanbul, Turkey; 2023. pp. 2449–57. https://doi.org/10.1109/BIBM58861.2023.10385256.

Suggestions for APA Research and Translational Perspective

5

This chapter is not intended for an in-depth exploration of a topic that falls within the expertise of trained computer scientists and other professionals. Its purpose is to offer insights and suggestions for applying their knowledge to research in the field of pain medicine.

5.1 Pain Glossary

To optimize the shared research processes in the field of AI applied to pain, bioinformaticians, engineers, and computer scientists must confront a complex set of phenomena, clinical conditions, and therapies. Fragmentation is not uncommon, for example, regarding background and breakthrough cancer pain or different types of pain, leading to errors in the feature engineering phase. To facilitate a common understanding and improve interdisciplinary collaboration, a glossary of definitions and practical terminologies is provided below.

Pain: the IASP Definition: According to the International Association for the Study of Pain (IASP), pain is "An unpleasant sensory and emotional experience associated with, or resembling that associated with, actual or potential tissue damage." It is a subjective feeling and can vary greatly in intensity and type [1].

Nociception is the sensory process by which harmful or potentially harmful stimuli are detected by the nervous system, leading to the perception of pain. It involves the activation of specialized sensory receptors called nociceptors. In other words, nociception is the complex neural process that enables the detection and response to potentially harmful stimuli, forming the basis for the experience of pain. The latter is a subjective experience that arises from the brain's interpretation of nociceptive signals. Therefore, pain is an emotional and sensory experience that is influenced by various factors, including psychological, emotional, and contextual elements [2].

© The Author(s), under exclusive license to Springer Nature Switzerland AG 2024
M. Cascella, *Exploring AI in Pain Research and Management*, https://doi.org/10.1007/978-3-031-78833-8_5

Nociceptors: They are specialized sensory neurons located throughout the body, particularly in the skin, joints, muscles, and internal organs. They detect thermal, mechanical, and chemical stimuli that may cause tissue damage.

Nerve fibers: Pain sensations are transmitted through different types of nerve fibers, each with distinct characteristics. The first type, A-alpha fibers, have a diameter of about 13–20 μm and conduct signals at a speed of 80–120 m/s. They are responsible for transmitting information related to position and spatial awareness. The second type, A-beta fibers, have a diameter of 6–13 μm and carry touch signals at a speed of 35–75 m/s. A-delta fibers, the third type, have a smaller diameter of about 1–5 μm and a slower conduction speed of 5–35 m/s. Despite this, they transmit information related to sharp pain and temperature. The last type, C fibers, are the smallest, with a diameter of 0.2–1.5 μm, and have the slowest conduction speed, ranging from 0.5–2.0 m/s. These fibers carry information about dull pain, temperature, and itching. The varying speeds of these fibers can result in a sequential sensation of pain. For instance, when someone pricks their finger, they first experience a sharp pain due to the faster A-delta fibers, followed by a slower, dull ache carried by the C fibers. This is partly because A-delta fibers are larger and myelinated, allowing for quicker signal transmission.

Pain Threshold: The point at which a stimulus begins to be perceived as painful.

Pain Tolerance: The maximum level of pain that a person is willing to tolerate.

Autonomic nervous system (ANS): It regulates involuntary bodily functions, ensuring that processes such as heart rate, digestion, respiratory rate, and blood pressure occur without conscious effort. The ANS operates through a continuous balance of two main branches: the sympathetic and parasympathetic nervous systems, which have complementary but opposing effects. The sympathetic nervous system is often referred to as the "fight or flight" system. It prepares the body for stressful or emergency situations. When activated, it increases heart rate, dilates pupils, relaxes airways, and inhibits digestion. This allows the body to respond quickly to perceived threats by mobilizing energy and redirecting blood flow to muscles and vital organs. In contrast, the parasympathetic nervous system (also known as the "rest and digest" system) promotes relaxation and recovery by slowing the heart rate, constricting pupils, stimulating digestion, and encouraging energy storage. Therefore, this ANS branch helps the body conserve energy and maintain homeostasis after a stressful event.

Acute Pain: It is a type of pain that typically lasts for a short duration, usually less than 3–6 months. It often occurs suddenly due to injury, surgery (postoperative pain), or illness and is typically sharp or intense.

Chronic Pain: It is pain that persists for longer than 3–6 months, often beyond the expected period of healing. It can be continuous or intermittent and may vary in intensity. Notably, chronic pain may not have a clear cause or persist after the initial cause has healed. While acute pain usually responds well to treatment aimed at the underlying cause, chronic pain often requires a more comprehensive management approach.

Chronic pain is classified in the International Classification of Diseases 11th Revision (ICD-11) as either primary or secondary [3]. *Chronic primary pain* has no clear underlying condition that sufficiently explains the pain or its impact. Fibromyalgia is a typical disease of chronic primary pain. In contrast, *chronic secondary pain* is associated with an identifiable underlying condition. Examples of chronic secondary pain conditions are cancer-related pain, and chronic low back pain.

Peripheral sensitization refers to the increased sensitivity of nociceptors (pain receptors) in the peripheral nervous system. This heightened sensitivity typically occurs after an injury or inflammation, leading to an exaggerated response to stimuli (e.g., in arthritis, where inflammation causes joint pain sensitivity).

Central sensitization involves increased responsiveness of neurons in the central nervous system to normal or subthreshold afferent input. This phenomenon is often associated with chronic pain conditions and is characterized by an amplification of pain signals in the spinal cord and brain.

Nociceptive Pain: Acute or chronic pain caused by damage to body tissue. Nociceptive pain has two subtypes: somatic pain which originates from skin, muscles, bones, or joints and visceral pain which originates from internal organs. The former (somatic pain) is typically localized and may be sharp or aching, visceral pain is often described as deep, squeezing, or cramping.

Neuropathic Pain: This pain is caused by damage or disease affecting the somatosensory nervous system (centrally or peripherally). It is often described as burning, shooting, or stabbing.

Nociplastic Pain: The term refers to pain that arises from altered nociception despite no clear evidence of actual or threatened tissue damage causing the activation of peripheral nociceptors or evidence of disease or lesion of the somatosensory system causing the pain. This type of pain is thought to result from a dysfunction in the way the nervous system processes pain signals, leading to an enhanced or abnormal pain perception. It is featured by central sensitization, diffuse pain, absence of clear pathology, enhanced pain sensitivity with *hyperalgesia* (increased pain from a stimulus that normally provokes pain) and *allodynia* (pain from stimuli that do not normally provoke pain). Examples are fibromyalgia and irritable bowel syndrome.

Breakthrough cancer pain (BTcP) refers to a transient and severe episode of pain that occurs despite otherwise well-controlled, chronic background pain in cancer patients. This type of pain "breaks through" the regular pain management regimen and can be challenging to manage. This cancer-related pain can be spontaneous or triggered by movements or other conditions [4, 5].

Pain Assessment: Is the process of evaluating the intensity, quality, and location of pain using scales (like the visual analog scale or numeric rating scale) and questionnaires. SOCRATES (i.e., Site. Onset, Character, Radiation, Associated symptoms, Time course, Exacerbating/relieving factors, and.

Severity) is a structured framework often used to assess pain?

Analgesics: Medications specifically designed to relieve pain. They include non-opioid analgesics such as acetaminophen and nonsteroidal anti-inflammatory drugs (NSAIDs) like ibuprofen, and opioid analgesics such as morphine, oxycodone, and hydrocodone, fentanyl.

Adjuvant analgesics are medications like antidepressants and anticonvulsants that can help manage certain types of pain, particularly neuropathic pain.

Opioid Tolerance: A phenomenon where increasing doses of opioids are needed to achieve the same level of pain relief due to the body's adaptation to the drug.

Opioid Use Disorder: Clinical condition characterized by a problematic pattern of opioid use leading to significant impairment of the patient's daily life or distress. It involves both a physical dependence on opioids and a behavioral pattern of misuse featuring loss of control, craving, and opioid use despite negative consequences.

Non-pharmacological treatments are a set of approaches useful as unique therapy or, more often, within a multimodal analgesic pathway [6]. These treatments include physical therapy, psychological approaches, acupuncture, transcutaneous or percutaneous electrical nerve stimulation, spinal cord stimulation, and other techniques [7].

Neuromodulation: It involves using technology to influence the neural interface and modulate the function of the central, peripheral, or autonomic nervous systems. This process includes the electrical or chemical stimulation, inhibition, modification, or regulation of neural activity for therapeutic purposes.

5.2 Suggestions for Crossing the AI Chasm

Interdisciplinary collaboration between computer scientists, clinicians, and other researchers is essential for the successful implementation of AI in pain assessment and management. Clinicians bring in-depth knowledge of patient care, pain physiology, and the clinical workflow, while computer scientists contribute expertise in AI methodologies, data analytics, and software development. One of the best practices for fostering such collaboration is establishing multidisciplinary teams that include data scientists, healthcare providers, and bioinformaticians from the project's inception. The close collaboration facilitates the exchange of ideas and ensures that all team members are aligned on objectives and methodologies. This approach is of paramount importance and helps bridge the gap between clinical needs and technical capabilities. The term "AI chasm" refers to the gap between the current limitations and capabilities of AI systems and the potential benefits that could be realized with more advanced technologies [8]. This gap acts as a barrier, hindering the full integration of AI into many real-world applications and creating a disparity between the hype surrounding AI and its actual capabilities. For instance, an analysis in the US found that only 14% of research findings make their way into clinical practice within 17 years [9]. Consequently, bridging the AI chasm is a significant challenge for the future of AI development [10]. In this scenario, clinicians provide insights into relevant clinical variables, indicate outcomes, and validate the model's predictions, while computer scientists optimize the algorithms and manage data preprocessing.

Practically, collaboration needs to be close to optimize both the preprocessing phase and the exploratory one. During these stages, effective communication and coordination between the clinician, computer scientist, and bioengineer are crucial. Elements that might appear minor or negligible to any one of these professionals can have a substantial impact on the modeling process. For instance, specific clinical elements, technical details, or engineering considerations could significantly influence the outcome of the model.

More importantly, to maximize the benefits of AI technologies, it is crucial to provide education and training for both computer scientists and clinicians. For computer scientists, understanding the clinical aspects of the research is fundamental. In the field of pain medicine, this includes learning about pain physiology, the various types of pain, patient assessment methods, and the specific challenges faced in clinical settings. This strategy is crucial to enable them to design AI models that are not only technically sound but also clinically meaningful. Training programs such as workshops, seminars by medical professionals, academic courses, and case studies can be highly beneficial. In parallel, clinicians should be trained on the basics of AI and its applications in healthcare. This includes an introduction to machine learning concepts, data analytics, and the interpretation of AI model outputs. This process can also help in overcoming the skepticism towards the reliability of AI in healthcare [11].

5.3 Suggestions for a Dashboard

In a research framework focused on APA, it is crucial to gather a comprehensive set of multimodal information. This includes physiological data, audiovisual materials such as video diaries, and questionnaires assessing pain and quality of life as well as other variables such as demographics and therapy. All this data must be systematically stored in a database to optimize both writing and reading operations.

To maximize the utility of this data, a user-friendly graphical interface is thus indispensable. Such an interface can easily allow researchers to efficiently navigate and utilize the collected information. Notably, in APA research, the platform can allow real-time monitoring.

Given its required functioning, this tool must balance completeness with simplicity, ensuring that it is both robust and easy to use. According to Gröger et al. [12], a dashboard is a panel that consolidates information from various visual resources, such as graphs and maps, which can be integrated to monitor, analyze, and facilitate decision-making across all hierarchical levels. Since up to 80% of the human brain is dedicated to visual processing—encompassing vision, memory, colors, shapes, movement, patterns, spatial awareness, and image recall—data visualization is a crucial step. It leverages the brain's ability to recognize patterns, thereby accelerating data comprehension [13]. Thus, dashboard development is a crucial aspect of the research.

Defining the requirements for the data visualization dashboard involves specifying both functional and non-functional prerequisites. Functional requirements cover what the dashboard should do, such as data integration, visualization capabilities, and user interaction features (Table 5.1). Non-functional requirements address the

Table 5.1 Example of functional requirements for APA research

Log in to the dashboard
Log out
View the list of patients registered on the platform
View the summary patient's information
View the history of the collected data
Pain scores (e.g., NRS) entered
Vital signs collected
Recorded video diaries
Completed questionnaires
Acute crisis reports (e.g., breakthrough cancer pain)
Other activities entered
View the patient's current therapy
Assign a new therapy to a patient
View the list of drugs on the platform
Insert, modify, or delete a drug

quality attributes of the dashboard, such as performance, usability, reliability, and scalability. Together, these prerequisites ensure that the dashboard will be an effective tool for managing and analyzing the multimodal information within the APA research framework.

Regarding non-functional prerequisites, the dashboard could be developed as a web app. This eliminates the need for software installation and allows quick access from any device with an internet browser. Additionally, the web app can be optimized for different screen sizes while maintaining a user interface designed primarily for desktop and tablet views. The system must ensure an acceptable startup time and responsive search functionality.

High-fidelity mock-ups represent software in the advanced stages of design. They surpass placeholders and wireframe "lorem ipsum" by incorporating actual content, fonts, colors, images, and branding. During the interface creation, every decision must meticulously align with established principles of user experience design. For this aim, it is possible to follow Shneiderman's eight golden rules of interface design [14] and Nielsen's ten heuristics [15], aiming to ensure the dashboard's clarity and user-friendliness.

Shneiderman's Golden Rules:

1. Strive for consistency.
2. Seek universal usability.
3. Offer informative feedback.
4. Design dialogs to yield closure.
5. Prevent errors.
6. Permit easy reversal of actions.
7. Keep users in control.
8. Reduce short-term memory load.

For example, to maintain consistency (Rule 1), it is suggested to use a light blue color scheme for most clickable elements and confirmation buttons. To prevent user errors such as omitting a dosage when adding a drug to the therapy (Rule 5), the system displays a prompt reminding the user to input the required dose.

Nielsen's Usability Heuristics principles:

1. Visibility of system status.
2. Match between the system and the real world.
3. User control and freedom.
4. Consistency and standards.
5. Error prevention.
6. Recognition rather than recall.
7. Flexibility and efficiency of use.
8. Aesthetic and minimalist design.
9. Help users recognize, diagnose, and recover from errors.
10. Help and documentation.

For instance, when an operator adds a drug to the therapy but later decides to remove it, a red "X" icon near the list of drugs allows easy removal, adhering to Principle 3. Additionally, the design embraces minimalism (Principle 8) by including only essential elements in each window. To simplify data entry, it is possible to add "hints" within text fields that disappear when the user begins typing and reappear if the text is cleared, enhancing usability.

The last step is the usability assessment. It measures how effectively and efficiently users achieve specific objectives with the system while deriving satisfaction from the process. The assessment involves various activities depending on the method used, with common methods including data acquisition, data analysis, and critique.

Usability refers to how effectively, efficiently, and satisfactorily a user can interact with a product, system, or service to achieve their goals. It is a crucial aspect of user experience (UX) design, ensuring that products are user-friendly and meet the needs of their intended users. According to Nielsen, usability is defined by five quality attributes including learning, efficiency, memory, error, and satisfaction [16]. Usability tests are typically divided into two macro-categories: task tests and scenario tests. Task tests involve users performing individual tasks that exercise multiple system functions, simulating real situations. These tests are valuable as they reflect actual user experiences, allowing us to understand if, where, and why users face challenges. Although users are focused on achieving a specific goal, they are not informed about the intermediate steps needed, making task tests a realistic measure of usability.

5.4 Useful Pain Databases

Data mining is the process used for extracting features and patterns (e.g., EEG recording) from large databases. It implements statistical methods, machine learning, and other AI-related fields. For the study of automatic pain assessment with AI, the availability of datasets is essential to train models on high-quality datasets with characteristics that align with the study's objectives. For example, linguistic analysis faces the main obstacles consisting of the scarcity of data available for training models and the need to reference datasets that align with the research objectives. A typical example of a biased source is found in the study of facial expressions for automatic pain assessment. Most of the research in this area has been conducted in Western countries, which may result in the underrepresentation of the Asian population. Although some datasets include Asian individuals, these studies primarily focus on physical differences, often neglecting the cultural and institutional factors that are crucial in healthcare [17].

Several databases can be used for APA research.

- BioVid Heat Pain Database [18]. Ninety participants underwent experimentally induced heat pain at four different intensities. To account for individual differences in heat pain sensitivity, stimulation temperatures were tailored to each participant's specific pain threshold and pain tolerance. Each of the four pain levels was administered 20 times in a randomized sequence. The peak temperature for each stimulus was maintained for 4 s, with intervals between stimuli ranging randomly from 8 to 12 s. The pain stimulation experiment was performed twice: once with the participants' faces unobstructed and once with facial EMG sensors in place.
- VGGFace2. Includes facial expression ($n = 9000$) from healthy subjects [19].
- The UNBC-McMaster Shoulder Pain dataset comprises video recordings of 129 participants (66 females and 63 males) experiencing shoulder pain. These recordings document active and passive range-of-motion tests conducted on both the affected and unaffected limbs across two distinct sessions. During the sessions, certified FACS coders analyzed and rated the AU intensity for each frame of the participants' facial expressions. In addition to the video data, the dataset includes self-reported pain levels and observer assessments collected at the sequence level, reflecting both the participants' subjective pain experiences and the researchers' observations. There are 200 spontaneous pain video sequences with 48,398 frames [20].
- The Delaware Pain Database is a collection of photos depicting painful expressions. To create this repository, 240 individuals (127 females and 113 males) were photographed first with neutral facial expressions and then displaying their reactions to five potentially painful scenarios. Each scenario included various levels of pain. The collected images were then processed by rating emotional features and applying the FACS. Ultimately, the researchers selected 229 unique images of painful expressions [21].

- Medical Speech database. It contains 8.5 h of audio utterances paired with text for common medical symptoms [22].
- BP4D-Spontaneous Database. It contains facial expressions and head poses collected from 41 healthy subjects [23].
- SenseEmotion Database. A multimodal sensory data including biopotentials, camera images of the facial region, and audio signals collected from 45 healthy individuals [24].
- Multimodal iIntensity Pain (MIntPAIN). Facial expressions collected from 20 healthy subjects [25].
- EmoPain. It is a multimodal dataset from University College London, comprising face videos, audio recordings, and electromyographic signals from back muscles of chronic pain patients [26].
- EMOVO. This emotional corpus (in Italian) was built from the voices of up to six actors who played 14 sentences simulating six emotional states (disgust, fear, anger, joy, surprise, sadness) plus the neutral state [27].
- UK Data Service UK database. Cortical, behavioral, and physiological responses were collected in neonates [28].
- The infant Classification of Pain Expression (iCOPE) dataset comprises 204 color images of 26 Caucasian infants, half girls, captured using a Nikon D100 digital camera. The infants, ranging in age from hours to days and all in good health, were photographed while exposed to four different stimuli: a pain stimulus during heel lancing (60 images), a rest/cry stimulus during transportation from one crib to another (63 rest images and 18 cry images), an air stimulus to the nose (23 images), and a friction stimulus involving the application of alcohol-soaked cotton to the external lateral surface of the heel (36 images) [29, 30].
- UNIFESP Image Dataset. Developed by Heiderich et al. [31] at the Federal University of São Paulo, the UNIFESP dataset includes 30 healthy neonates (7 late preterm and 23 full-term) with gestational ages between 34 and 41 weeks and ages ranging from 24 to 168 h. For each neonate, 10-min videos were recorded before, during, and after painful procedures like venipuncture, capillary puncture, and intramuscular injection, performed during routine tests or vaccine administration. Images were extracted from these videos every 3 s.

Other databases can be found in different repositories such as Zenodo, where we collected different databases containing multimodal data [32, 33].

5.5 Wearable Health-Monitoring Systems and Devices for APA

Wearable Health Monitoring Systems (WHMS) and other tools used for biosignal or behavioral research play a crucial role in APA investigations [34–64]. Within the research frameworks, they are selected based on different aspects. Their ability to seamlessly integrate into patients' daily lives, for instance, is an important feature.

The device's ease of use and its capability to accurately extract physiological signals for processing including the limitations related to copyright, are paramount elements that require careful evaluation.

A WHMS consists of multiple components, including sensors, wearable materials, smart textiles, power supplies, communication modules, a central processing unit (CPU), software, and advanced algorithms. For practical application, these systems must meet several criteria, such as being lightweight and compact for enhanced comfort, ensuring low radiation and minimal heat dissipation for safety, and maintaining appropriate security during data transmission to address privacy concerns. Additionally, the overall system must be cost-effective and affordable, even for underprivileged populations.

Their maturity level refers to the system's ability to measure multiple parameters, the level of detail in data documentation, the system's popularity (measured by citation count), the hardware technologies used, and the algorithms employed for feature extraction and, eventually, decision support [61]. Notably, even systems with the highest maturity levels must address challenges such as limited battery life and the security of private information.

By integrating modern technologies like cloud computing and fog computing, WHMS can enhance performance while minimizing the cost of electronic components and processing units, and freeing up space for additional sensors. Such integrations offload heavy computing tasks from the data collection unit, reducing power consumption and freeing up sensor capacity [62]. Additionally, using smartphones as data transmission and processing hubs can create a more comprehensive and compatible platform [63]. Federated learning can then transform explicit data into implicit data, reducing the risk of data leakage and speeding up the optimization of diagnostic models.

Devices for recording behavior offer complex functionality but have the advantage of being able to integrate with multiple other devices including WHMSs, for developing a comprehensive platform. For example, Next2U's Hybrid InfraRed System for Affective Computing (HIRA) system classifies six predefined facial expressions directly from facial images with an accuracy of 70%. The system outputs are all in text/numeric format, meaning the results are published as text values on an output port. By connecting to this port, the results can be read in real time and used according to the specific use case. Alternatively, the data can also be saved as text files or CSV tables. Integrated systems include respiratory rate (numeric value and classification into bradypnea, tachypnea, or normal rate), autonomic dominance (binary value classifying sympathetic or parasympathetic dominance), perspiration level (three-level classification: absent, low, high), thermal engagement (six-class classification based on the circumplex model of emotions), and thermal comfort (cold, normal, hot) [64].

Table 5.2 includes a mix of sensors that are either directly or indirectly used for pain assessment.

Table 5.2 Selected commercialized wearable sensors used for biosignal investigations and behavioral investigations

Type of Signal/Aim	Wearable Device(s) [Ref.]
Wearable health–monitoring systems	
Heart activity	Bitalino [34, 48], Empatica E4 wristband [43], AutoSense [47], BioHarness 3 [40], Wahoo chest belt [46], DataLOG [39, 54]
Brain activity (EEG)	Bitalino [48], MindWave Mobile EEG headset [40], Muse Headband [49], Emotiv Epoc+ [50], Enobio 8 [60]
Muscle activity (EMG and sEMG)	Bitalino [34], Myo armband [51], DataLOG [39], Delsys Trigno [53]
Electrodermal activity (EDA)	Bitalino [34], Empatica E4 wristband [42], Affectiva Q-sensor [35], Shimmer sensor [40], BioHarness [40], 3 BN-PPGED [38]
Respiratory	BioHarness 3 [40], AutoSense [47]
Blood volume pulse/pulse plethysmograph	Empatica E4 wristband [42, 44, 45], BN-PPGED [38], Polar H10 [53]
Body/skin temperature	Empatica E4 wristband [45], AutoSense [47], iButton [55], BioHarness 3 [40]
Three-axis accelerometer data	Bitalino [34, 48], Empatica E4 wristband [45], Affectiva Q-sensor [36, 37], ActiGraph GT9X [58]
Devices	
Facial expression analysis (camera)	RealSense Depth Camera [57], Affectiva Affdex SDK [59]
Vocal analysis (affective computing)	Beyond Verbal [41], Sonde Health [56]
Multi-feature analysis (affective computing)	Next2U HIRA [64]

5.6 A Suggested Research Framework

A comprehensive framework for APA integrates various components to create a robust system for personalized pain management. The framework begins with patient interaction, where pain is assessed through both quantitative and qualitative methods. Standard qualitative assessment involves subjective methods like self-reporting, questionnaires, and clinical evaluations to capture the patient's pain experience. Unimodal scales and multidimensional tools can be implemented.

In contrast, quantitative assessment relies on objective measurement techniques, such as biosignal recordings and behavioral analysis, to quantify pain levels. Behavioral strategies, including facial expression analysis, verbal analysis, and speech emotion recognition capture different indicators of pain, such as facial muscle movements. They also analyze speech patterns to detect emotional states like stress or anxiety, which are often linked to pain. Alongside these strategies, a wearable multisignal platform plays a crucial role in continuously monitoring the patient's physiological signals, such as heart rate and skin conductance.

Central to the framework is a dashboard for data recording and visualization, integrating inputs from wearable devices, behavioral analysis tools, and AI algorithms. This dashboard would provide healthcare providers with a comprehensive

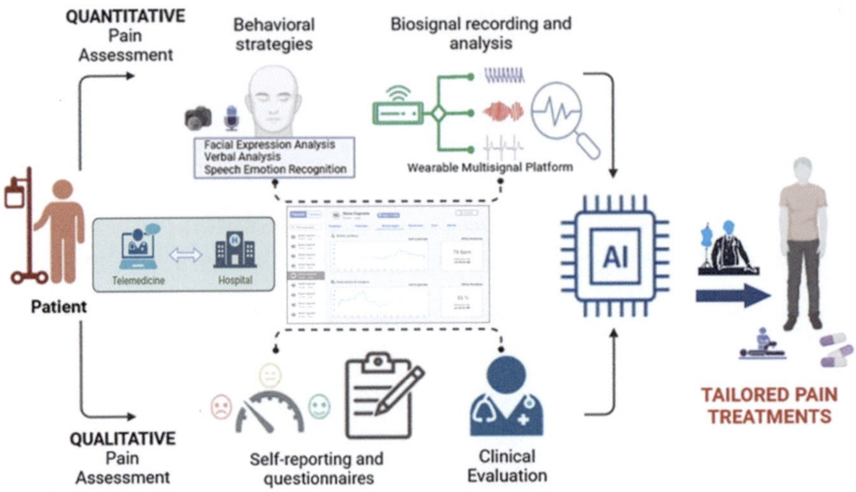

Fig. 5.1 A holistic approach to pain assessment, combining advanced technology with traditional methods to offer a personalized and responsive solution for pain management

view of the patient's pain status. It can also enable remote monitoring, treatment adjustments, and timely responses to significant changes, offering real-time data that is essential for accurate pain assessment.

The integration of telemedicine can be a key element of the framework. This connection between the patient and the hospital enables continuous monitoring and real-time data sharing, allowing healthcare providers to access both live and historical data for informed decision-making.

Different AI strategies are employed to process the collected data, identify patterns, and predict pain levels. The output of this framework is tailored pain treatments, developed from the AI-driven analysis and combined quantitative and qualitative assessments. In more advanced frameworks, a feedback loop can provide a process where the outcomes of tailored treatments are continuously fed back into the system, refining the pain assessment algorithms and improving the overall efficacy of pain management over time. This iterative process can ensure that the system remains adaptive, becoming increasingly accurate and effective in addressing individual patient needs (Fig. 5.1).

5.7 Automatic Pain Recognition in Animals

Pain is not exclusive to humans. Recognizing and effectively addressing pain in animals is a crucial aspect of veterinary medicine and animal welfare. Unlike humans, animals cannot verbally communicate their discomfort, making identifying and assessing pain particularly challenging. Consequently, undetected, or untreated pain can lead to prolonged suffering, compromised recovery, and diminished overall quality of life for animals. This issue is especially pertinent in both clinical and research settings, where accurate pain assessment is essential for appropriate treatment decisions and ethical research practices [65], maintaining ethical standards and ensuring the welfare of animals involved in studies. Therefore, failure to recognize and alleviate pain in research animals not only compromises their well-being but also impairs the validity and reliability of experimental results [66]. In laboratory settings and different animal models, indeed, precise pain assessment is mandatory for the translation of results [67]. On these bases, developing reliable and objective methods for pain recognition in animals is imperative for advancing both veterinary medicine and scientific research as well as for aiding animal caretakers.

Although physiological and behavioral can be adopted for the aim, in animals, behavioral pain assessment is preferred due to its non-intrusive, non-invasive, and cost-effective nature [68]. For detecting pain in laboratory animals researchers can use "traditional" behavioral methods, such as weight loss or head movements and postures [69]. Nevertheless, this strategy has no reproducibility and is not accurate to promptly intercept pain.

Similarly to humans, changes in facial expressions offer a reliable and rapid method for assessing pain in animals. Key elements for the analysis are the action units (AUs) that represent the expression of involuntary facial muscle movements. In 1978, psychologists Paul Ekman and Wallace V. Friesen developed the Facial Action Coding System (FACS) to analyze and catalog human facial expressions (i.e., AUs) and attribute psychological significance [70]. A set of recognized AUs has been used for objective pain investigations [71, 72].

The Grimace Scale is an AU-based behavioral pain assessment method that relies on observing and interpreting facial expressions and subtle changes in facial features, such as eye squinting, ear position, and changes in the position and shape of whisker, to infer the presence and intensity of pain. This approach was first developed to evaluate pain in mice [73]. Subsequently, various versions of the Grimace Scale have been tailored to different species for assessing pain in laboratory animals and veterinary medicine [74]. The feline grimace scale, for example, was developed for the objective assessment of pain in cats [75] and other scales were validated in horses [76], and sheep [77]. Behavior-based methods relying on facial expressions have been also investigated in pigs [78].

Similarly to Ekman's Facial Action Coding System FLACS for humans, manual assessment of AUs in scales for animals may require complex training of the operator [68]. Furthermore, in some species, the systems, and associations of AUs with other parameters are not well codified [78]. Moreover, these manual approaches may be effective in identifying acute pain phenomena such as procedural pain, but they do not adequately address chronic pain. Most importantly, these systems do not facilitate continuous pain monitoring as they rely on relatively short observational time windows. Given that pain often occurs episodically or fluctuates in intensity, continuous monitoring is essential to avoid missing critical pain events [79].

Facial expressions are not the sole potential means to study pain in animals. For instance, in pigs, the Unesp-Botucatu Pig Composite Acute Pain Scale (UPAPS) was validated to diagnose pain using a combination of six behavioral items

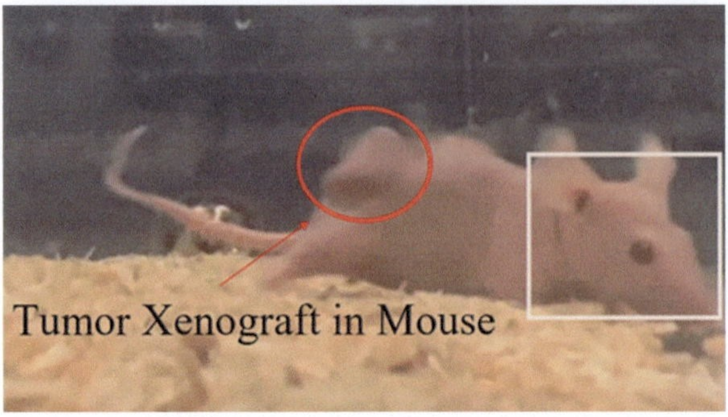

Fig. 5.2 Automatic pain assessment in mouse. Experimental animal with a xenograft tumor (triple-negative breast cancer cell lines). The compression of the mass (indicated by the red circle) likely induces pain, possibly neuropathic pain due to nerve compression. A high-resolution camera records facial expressions for automatic pain assessment. From the author

including posture, interaction and interest in the surroundings, activity, appetite, attention, and other grouped behaviors. Four score levels: "0," "1," "2," and "3" are assigned according to the type of pain-related behavior [80].

In recent years, advances in technology, particularly in the field of AI, have offered promising opportunities for improving pain recognition and assessment in animals. AI-based approaches have the potential to analyze complex data patterns and identify subtle indicators of pain that may not be readily apparent to human observers. This field of research is referred to as automatic pain assessment (APA) [81]. Several efforts have been made to apply AI techniques for studying pain through grimace scales in mice [82], cats [83], and pigs [84–86].

The research process closely mirrors the methodology used in human studies. Initially, a model is constructed, typically a neural network designed for computer vision tasks. This model is then trained using a comprehensive reference dataset that contains labeled examples of the target phenomena, such as facial expressions indicating pain. The typical steps: image preprocessing, feature extraction, and classification can be implemented. Once the training phase is complete, the model's performance is rigorously evaluated using validation techniques to ensure its accuracy and reliability. Only after these steps are completed, the model is tested in real world or experimental settings to assess its practical applicability and effectiveness (Fig. 5.2).

References

1. Raja SN, Carr DB, Cohen M, Finnerup NB, Flor H, Gibson S, Keefe FJ, Mogil JS, Ringkamp M, Sluka KA, Song XJ, Stevens B, Sullivan MD, Tutelman PR, Ushida T, Vader K. The revised International Association for the Study of Pain definition of pain: concepts, challenges, and compromises. Pain. 2020;161(9):1976–82. https://doi.org/10.1097/j.pain.0000000000001939.
2. Cascella M, Muzio MR, Monaco F, Nocerino D, Ottaiano A, Perri F, Innamorato MA. Pathophysiology of nociception and rare genetic disorders with increased pain thresh-

old or pain insensitivity. Pathophysiology. 2022;29(3):435–52. https://doi.org/10.3390/pathophysiology29030035.
3. Treede R-D, Rief W, Barke A, Aziz Q, Bennett MI, Benoliel R, et al. Chronic pain as a symptom or a disease: the IASP classification of chronic pain for the international classification of diseases (ICD-11) pain United States. Pain. 2019;160:19–27.
4. Bossi P, Pietrzyńska T, Margarit Ferri C, Mansilla I, Tellone V, Fioravanti S, Di Loreto G, Comandini A. Compliance with the breakthrough cancer pain European guidelines and impact on patients' quality of life: an observational prospective study. Front Pain Res (Lausanne). 2024;5:1388837. https://doi.org/10.3389/fpain.2024.1388837.
5. Portenoy RK, Bruns D, Shoemaker B, Shoemaker SA. Breakthrough pain in community-dwelling patients with cancer pain and noncancer pain, part 1: prevalence and characteristics. J Opioid Manag. 2010;6(2):97–108. https://doi.org/10.5055/jom.2010.0009.
6. Cuomo A, Bimonte S, Forte CA, Botti G, Cascella M. Multimodal approaches and tailored therapies for pain management: the trolley analgesic model. J Pain Res. 2019;12:711–4. https://doi.org/10.2147/JPR.S178910.
7. Monaco F, Coluccia S, Cuomo A, Nocerino D, Schiavo D, Pasta G, Bifulco F, Buonanno P, Riccio V, Leonardi M, et al. Bibliometric and visual analysis of the scientific literature on percutaneous electrical nerve stimulation (PENS) for pain treatment. Appl Sci. 2023;13(1):636. https://doi.org/10.3390/app13010636.
8. Aristidou A, Jena R, Topol EJ. Bridging the chasm between AI and clinical implementation. Lancet. 2022;399:620.
9. Westfall JM, Mold J, Fagnan L. Practice-based research—"blue highways" on the NIH roadmap. JAMA. 2007;297:403–6.
10. Car J, Sheikh A, Wicks P, Williams MS. Beyond the hype of big data and artificial intelligence: building foundations for knowledge and wisdom. BMC Med. 2019;17:143.
11. Cascella M, Montomoli J, Bellini V, Vittori A, Biancuzzi H, Dal Mas F, Bignami EG. Crossing the AI chasm in neurocritical care. Computers. 2023;12(4):83. https://doi.org/10.3390/computers12040083.
12. Gröger C, Hillmann M, Hahn F, Mitschang B, Westkämper E. The operational process dashboard for manufacturing. Proc CIRP. 2013;7:205–10. https://doi.org/10.1016/j.procir.2013.05.035.
13. Matheus R, Janssen M, Maheshwari D. Data science empowering the public: data-driven dashboards for transparent and accountable decision-making in smart cities. Gov Inf Q. 2020;37(3):101284. https://doi.org/10.1016/j.giq.2018.01.006.
14. Shneiderman B, Plaisant C, Cohen M, Jacobs S, Elmqvist N, Diakopoulos N. Designing the user Interface: strategies for effective human-computer interaction, Global Edition. Sixth ed. Pearson Education; 2018.
15. Nielsen J. Enhancing the explanatory power of usability heuristics. In: Human factors in computing System; 1994.
16. Nielsen J. Usability 101: Introduction to usability. 2012. https://www.nngroup.com/articles/usability-101-introduction-to-usability/.
17. Gomutbutra P, Kittisares A, Sanguansri A, Choosri N, Sawaddiruk P, Fakfum P, Lerttrakarnnon P, Saralamba S. Classification of elderly pain severity from automated video clip facial action unit analysis: a study from a Thai data repository. Front Artif Intell. 2022;5:942248. https://doi.org/10.3389/frai.2022.942248.
18. Walter S, Gruss S, Ehleiter H. The biovid heat pain database data for the advancement and systematic val-idation of an automated pain recognition system. In: Cybernetics (CYBCONF) 2013 IEEE international conference on IEEE; 2013. p. 128–31.
19. Fernandez E, Vargas R, Mahometa M, Ramamurthy S, Boyle GJ. Descriptors of pain sensation: a dual hierarchical model of latent structure. J Pain. 2012;13(6):532–6. https://doi.org/10.1016/j.jpain.2012.02.006.
20. Lucey P, Cohn JF, Prkachin KM, Solomon PE, Matthews I. Painful data: the UNBC-McMaster shoulder pain expression archive database. In: 2011 IEEE International Conference on Automatic Face & Gesture Recognition (FG); 2011. p. 57–64.

21. Mende-Siedlecki P, Qu-Lee J, Lin J, Drain A, Goharzad A. The Delaware pain database: a set of painful expressions and corresponding norming data. Pain Rep. 2020;5:e853. https://doi.org/10.1097/PR9.0000000000000853.
22. Medical Speech Database. https://www.kaggle.com/datasets/paultimothymooney/medical-speech-transcription-and-intent/data. Accessed 2 Oct 2023.
23. Zhang X, Yin L, Cohn JF, et al. BP4D-spontaneous: a high-resolution spontaneous 3D dynamic facial expression database. Image Vis Comput. 2014;32(10):692–706. https://doi.org/10.1016/j.imavis.2014.06.002.
24. Velana M. The sense emotion database: a multimodal database for the development and systematic validation of an automatic pain-and emotion-recognition system. In: Schwenker F, Scherer S, editors. Multimodal pattern recognition of social signals in human-computer-interaction. MPRSS 2016. Lecture notes in computer science, vol. 10183. Cham: Springer; 2017.
25. Walter S, Al-Hamadi A, Gruss S, Frisch S, Traue HC, Werner P. Multimodale Erkennung von Schmerzintensität und-modalität mit maschinellen Lernverfahren [multimodal recognition of pain intensity and pain modality with machine learning]. Schmerz. 2020;34(5):400–9. https://doi.org/10.1007/s00482-020-00468-8.
26. Aung MSH, Kaltwang S, Romera-Paredes B, et al. The automatic detection of chronic pain-related expression: requirements, challenges and the multimodal EmoPain dataset. IEEE Trans Affect Comput. 2016;7(4):435–51. https://doi.org/10.1109/TAFFC.2015.2462830.
27. Costantini G, Iaderola I, Paoloni A, Todisco M. EMOVO corpus: an Italian emotional speech database. In: Proceedings of the ninth international conference on language resources and evaluation (LREC'14). Reykjavik: European Language Resources Association (ELRA); 2014. p. 3501–4.
28. UK Data Service UK database. https://ukdataservice.ac.uk/find-data/. Accessed 30 June 2024.
29. COPE Database. https://childrenofprisoners.eu/the-network/cope-database/. Accessed 30 June 2024.
30. Brahnam S, Chuang CF, Sexton RS, Shih FY. Machine assessment of neonatal facial expressions of acute pain. Decis Support Syst. 2007;43(4):1242–54.
31. Heiderich TM, Leslie AT, Guinsburg R. Neonatal procedural pain can be assessed by computer software that has good sensitivity and specificity to detect facial movements. Acta Paediatr. 2015;104(2):e63–9. https://doi.org/10.1111/apa.12861.
32. Cascella M. Dataset for binary Classifier_PAIN. 2023. https://doi.org/10.5281/zenodo.7557362.
33. Casella M. Corpus_PAIN [Data set]. Zenodo. 2023. https://doi.org/10.5281/zenodo.10060733.
34. Cascella M, Vitale VN, D'Antò M, Cuomo A, Amato F, Romano M, Ponsiglione AM. Exploring biosignals for quantitative pain assessment in cancer patients: a proof of concept. Electronics. 2023;12(17):3716. https://doi.org/10.3390/electronics12173716.
35. Bhatkar V, Picard R, Staahl C. Combining Electrodermal activity with the peak-pain time to quantify three temporal regions of pain experience. Front Pain Res (Lausanne). 2022;3:764128. https://doi.org/10.3389/fpain.2022.764128.
36. Ollander S, Godin C, Campagne A, Charbonnier S. A comparison of wearable and stationary sensors for stress detection. In: Proceedings of the 2016 IEEE international conference on systems, man, and cybernetics (SMC); Budapest, Hungary, 9–12 October 2016; 2016. p. 4362–6.
37. Sano A, Picard RW. Stress recognition using wearable sensors and Mobile phones. In: Proceedings of the 2013 Humaine association conference on affective computing and intelligent interaction; Geneva, Switzerland 2–5 September 2013; 2013. p. 671–6.
38. Sandulescu V, Andrews S, Ellis DA, Bellotto N, Mozos OM. Stress detection using wearable physiological sensors. In: Proceedings of international work-conference on the interplay between natural and artificial computation, vol. 1–5. Elche: IWINAC; 2015. p. 526–32.
39. Pourmohammadi S, Maleki A. Stress detection using ECG and EMG signals: a comprehensive study. Comput Methods Prog Biomed. 2020;193:105482. https://doi.org/10.1016/j.cmpb.2020.105482.
40. Betti S, Lova RM, Rovini E, Acerbi G, Santarelli L, Cabiati M, Del Ry S, Cavallo F. Evaluation of an integrated system of wearable physiological sensors for stress monitoring in work-

ing environments by using biological markers. IEEE Trans Biomed Eng. 2018;65:1748–58. https://doi.org/10.1109/tbme.2017.2764507.

41. Atis N, Dhillon R, Maichel V, Soto G, Vergara B. Beyond verbal: a low-cost communication tool to address language barriers in a community-based setting. Occup Ther Student Res. 2022;9:1.
42. Campanella S, Altaleb A, Belli A, Pierleoni P, Palma L. A method for stress detection using Empatica E4 bracelet and machine-learning techniques. Sensors (Basel). 2023;23(7):3565. https://doi.org/10.3390/s23073565.
43. Schuurmans AAT, de Looff P, Nijhof KS, Rosada C, Scholte RHJ, Popma A, Otten R. Validity of the Empatica E4 wristband to measure heart rate variability (HRV) parameters: a comparison to electrocardiography (ECG). J Med Syst. 2020;44(11):190. https://doi.org/10.1007/s10916-020-01648-w.
44. McCarthy C, Pradhan N, Redpath C, Adler A. Validation of the Empatica E4 wristband. In: 2016 IEEE EMBS international student conference (ISC), Ottawa, ON, Canada; 2016. p. 1–4. https://doi.org/10.1109/EMBSISC.2016.7508621.
45. Regalia G, Onorati F, Lai M, Caborni C, Picard RW. Multimodal wrist-worn devices for seizure detection and advancing research: focus on the Empatica wristbands. Epilepsy Res. 2019;153:79–82. https://doi.org/10.1016/j.eplepsyres.2019.02.007.
46. Muaremi A, Arnrich B, Tröster G. Towards measuring stress with smartphones and wearable devices during workday and sleep. BioNanoScience. 2013;3:172–83. https://doi.org/10.1007/s12668-013-0089-2.
47. Nakajima M, Lemieux AM, Fiecas M, Chatterjee S, Sarker H, Saleheen N, Ertin E, Kumar S, Al'Absi M. Using novel mobile sensors to assess stress and smoking lapse. Int J Psychophysiol. 2020;158:411–8. https://doi.org/10.1016/j.ijpsycho.2020.11.005.
48. Ponciano V, Pires IM, Ribeiro FR, Garcia NM. Data acquisition of timed-up and go test with older adults: accelerometer, magnetometer, electrocardiography and electroencephalography sensors' data. Data Brief. 2020;32:106306. https://doi.org/10.1016/j.dib.2020.106306.
49. Krigolson OE, Hammerstrom MR, Abimbola W, Trska R, Wright BW, Hecker KG, Binsted G. Using muse: rapid Mobile assessment of brain performance. Front Neurosci. 2021;15:634147. https://doi.org/10.3389/fnins.2021.634147.
50. Fouad IA. A robust and reliable online P300-based BCI system using Emotiv EPOC+headset. J Med Eng Technol. 2021;45(2):94–114. https://doi.org/10.1080/03091902.2020.1853840.
51. Marcos-Antón S, Gor-García-Fogeda MD, Cano-de-la-Cuerda R. An sEMG-controlled forearm bracelet for assessing and training manual dexterity in rehabilitation: a systematic review. J Clin Med. 2022;11(11):3119. https://doi.org/10.3390/jcm11113119.
52. Seo JW, Kang GH, Kim CH, Jung J, Kim J, Kang H, Lee S. Characteristics of gait event and muscle activation parameters of the lower limb on the affected side in patients with hemiplegia after stroke: a pilot study. Arch Rehab Res Clin Transl. 2023;5(4):100274. https://doi.org/10.1016/j.arrct.2023.100274.
53. Schaffarczyk M, Rogers B, Reer R, Gronwald T. Validity of the polar H10 sensor for heart rate variability analysis during resting state and incremental exercise in recreational men and women. Sensors (Basel). 2022;22(17):6536. https://doi.org/10.3390/s22176536.
54. Godino JG, Wing D, de Zambotti M, Baker FC, Bagot K, Inkelis S, Pautz C, Higgins M, Nichols J, Brumback T, Chevance G, Colrain IM, Patrick K, Tapert SF. Performance of a commercial multi-sensor wearable (Fitbit charge HR) in measuring physical activity and sleep in healthy children. PLoS One. 2020;15(9):e0237719. https://doi.org/10.1371/journal.pone.0237719.
55. Fawcett S, Sistla S, Dacosta-Calheiros M, Kahraman A, Reznicek AA, Rosenberg R, von Wettberg EJB. Tracking microhabitat temperature variation with iButton data loggers. Appl Plant Sci. 2019;7(4):e01237. https://doi.org/10.1002/aps3.1237.
56. Kaur S, Larsen E, Harper J, Purandare B, Uluer A, Hasdianda MA, Umale NA, Killeen J, Castillo E, Jariwala S. Development and validation of a respiratory-responsive vocal biomarker-based tool for generalizable detection of respiratory impairment: independent case-control

studies in multiple respiratory conditions including asthma, chronic obstructive pulmonary disease, and COVID-19. J Med Internet Res. 2023;25:e44410. https://doi.org/10.2196/44410.
57. Siena FL, Byrom B, Watts P, Breedon P. Utilising the Intel RealSense camera for measuring health outcomes in clinical research. J Med Syst. 2018;42(3):53. https://doi.org/10.1007/s10916-018-0905-x.
58. Suau Q, Bianchini E, Bellier A, Chardon M, Milane T, Hansen C, Vuillerme N. Current knowledge about ActiGraph GT9X link activity monitor accuracy and validity in measuring steps and energy expenditure: a systematic review. Sensors (Basel). 2024;24(3):825. https://doi.org/10.3390/s24030825.
59. Magdin M, Benko Ľ, Koprda Š. A case study of facial emotion classification using Affdex. Sensors (Basel). 2019;19(9):2140. https://doi.org/10.3390/s19092140.
60. Ratti E, Waninger S, Berka C, Ruffini G, Verma A. Comparison of medical and consumer wireless EEG Systems for use in clinical trials. Front Hum Neurosci. 2017;11:398. https://doi.org/10.3389/fnhum.2017.00398.
61. Pantelopoulos A, Bourbakis NG. A survey on wearable sensor-based Systems for Health Monitoring and Prognosis. IEEE Trans Syst Man Cybern Part C (Applications Rev). 2010;40:1–12. https://doi.org/10.1109/TSMCC.2009.2032660.
62. Chen J, Abbod MF, Shieh J-S. Integrations between autonomous systems and modern computing techniques: a mini review. Sensors. 2019;19:3897. https://doi.org/10.3390/s19183897.
63. Ozer E, Kromanis R. Smartphone prospects in bridge structural health monitoring, a literature review. Sensors (Basel). 2024;24(11):3287. https://doi.org/10.3390/s24113287.
64. Next2U HIRA. https://www.hira-project.com/. Accessed 24 June 2024.
65. Pritt SL, Hammer RE. The interplay of ethics, animal welfare, and IACUC oversight on the reproducibility of animal studies. Comp Med. 2017;67:101–5.
66. Carbone L. Pain in laboratory animals: the ethical and regulatory imperatives. PLoS One. 2011;6:e21578. https://doi.org/10.1371/journal.pone.0021578.
67. Lee KH, Lee DW, Kang BC. The 'R' principles in laboratory animal experiments. Lab Anim Res. 2020;36:45.
68. Aulehner K, Leenaars C, Buchecker V, Stirling H, Schönhoff K, King H, Häger C, Koska I, Jirkof P, Bleich A, Bankstahl M, Potschka H. Grimace scale, burrowing, and nest building for the assessment of post-surgical pain in mice and rats-a systematic review. Front Vet Sci. 2022;9:930005. https://doi.org/10.3389/fvets.2022.930005.
69. Werner P, Al-Hamadi A, Limbrecht-Ecklundt K, Walter S, Traue HC. Head movements and postures as pain behavior. PLoS One. 2018;13(2):e0192767. https://doi.org/10.1371/journal.pone.0192767.e0192767.
70. Ekman P, Friesen WV. Facial action coding system: Investigator's guide. Palo Alto, CA: Consulting Psychologists Press; 1978.
71. Hassan T, Seus D, Wollenberg J, Weitz K, Kunz M, Lautenbacher S, et al. Automatic detection of pain from facial expressions: a survey. IEEE Trans Pattern Anal Mach Intell. 2021;43:1815–31. https://doi.org/10.1109/TPAMI.2019.2958341.
72. Cascella M, Vitale VN, Mariani F, Iuorio M, Cutugno F. Development of a binary classifier model from extended facial codes toward video-based pain recognition in cancer patients. Scand J Pain. 2023;23(4):638–45. https://doi.org/10.1515/sjpain-2023-0011.
73. Langford DJ, Bailey AL, Chanda ML, Clarke SE, Drummond TE, Echols S, et al. Coding of facial expressions of pain in the laboratory mouse. Nat Methods. 2010;7:447–9.
74. Onuma K, Watanabe M, Sasaki N. The grimace scale: a useful tool for assessing pain in laboratory animals. Exp Anim. 2024;73:234. https://doi.org/10.1538/expanim.24-0010.
75. Evangelista MC, Watanabe R, Leung VSY, Monteiro BP, O'Toole E, Pang DSJ, et al. Facial expressions of pain in cats: the development and validation of a feline grimace scale. Sci Rep. 2019;9:19128.
76. Dalla Costa E, Minero M, Lebelt D, Stucke D, Canali E, Leach MC. Development of the horse grimace scale (HGS) as a pain assessment tool in horses undergoing routine castration. PLoS One. 2014;9:e92281.

77. McLennan K, Mahmoud M. Development of an automated pain facial expression detection system for sheep (Ovis Aries). Animals. 2019;9:196.
78. Di Giminiani P, Brierley VLMH, Scollo A, Gottardo F, Malcolm EM, Edwards SA, et al. The assessment of facial expressions in piglets undergoing tail docking and castration: toward the development of the piglet grimace scale. Front Vet Sci. 2016;3:100.
79. Lautenbacher S, Hassan T, Seuss D, Loy FW, Garbas JU, Schmid U, Kunz M. Automatic coding of facial expressions of pain: are we there yet? Pain Res Manag. 2022;2022:6635496. https://doi.org/10.1155/2022/6635496.
80. Luna SPL, et al. Validation of the UNESP-Botucatu pig composite acute pain scale (UPAPS). PLoS One. 2020;15:e0233552. https://doi.org/10.1371/journal.pone.0233552.
81. Cascella M, Schiavo D, Cuomo A, Ottaiano A, Perri F, Patrone R, Migliarelli S, Bignami EG, Vittori A, Cutugno F. Artificial intelligence for automatic pain assessment: research methods and perspectives. Pain Res Manag. 2023;6018736:6018736. https://doi.org/10.1155/2023/6018736.
82. Andresen N, Wöllhaf M, Hohlbaum K, Lewejohann L, Hellwich O, Thöne-Reineke C, Belik V. Towards a fully automated surveillance of Well-being status in laboratory mice using deep learning: starting with facial expression analysis. PLoS One. 2020;15(4):e0228059. https://doi.org/10.1371/journal.pone.0228059.
83. Steagall PV, Monteiro BP, Marangoni S, Moussa M, Sautié M. Fully automated deep learning models with smartphone applicability for prediction of pain using the feline grimace scale. Sci Rep. 2023;13(1):21584. https://doi.org/10.1038/s41598-023-49031-2.
84. Trindade PHE, de Araújo AL, Luna SPL. Weighted pain-related behaviors in pigs undergoing castration based on multilevel logistic regression algorithm. Appl Anim Behav Sci. 2023;265:106002. https://doi.org/10.1016/j.applanim.2023.106002.
85. da Silva GV, Pivato GM, Peres BG, Luna SPL, Pairis-Garcia MD, Trindade PHE. Simplified assessment of castration-induced pain in pigs using lower complexity algorithms. Sci Rep. 2023;13(1):21237. https://doi.org/10.1038/s41598-023-48551-1.
86. Robles I, Luna SPL, Trindade PHE, Lopez-Soriano M, Merenda VR, Viscardi AV, Tamminga E, Lou ME, Pairis-Garcia MD. Validation of the Unesp-Botucatu pig composite acute pain scale (UPAPS) in piglets undergoing castration. PLoS One. 2023;18:e0284218. https://doi.org/10.1371/journal.pone.0284218.

MIX
Papier aus verantwortungsvollen Quellen
Paper from responsible sources
FSC® C105338

FSC
www.fsc.org

If you have any concerns about our products,
you can contact us on
ProductSafety@springernature.com

In case Publisher is established outside the EU,
the EU authorized representative is:
Springer Nature Customer Service Center GmbH
Europaplatz 3, 69115 Heidelberg, Germany

Printed by Libri Plureos GmbH
in Hamburg, Germany